AVIATION SAFETY AND PILOT CONTROL

Understanding and Preventing Unfavorable Pilot-Vehicle Interactions

Committee on the Effects of Aircraft-Pilot Coupling on Flight Safety
Aeronautics and Space Engineering Board
Commission on Engineering and Technical Systems
National Research Council

NATIONAL ACADEMY PRESS
Washington, D.C. 1997

NOTICE: The project that is the subject of this report was approved by the Governing Board of the National Research Council, whose members are drawn from the councils of the National Academy of Sciences, the National Academy of Engineering, and the Institute of Medicine. The members of the panel responsible for the report were chosen for their special competencies and with regard for appropriate balance.

This report has been reviewed by a group other than the authors according to procedures approved by a Report Review Committee consisting of members of the National Academy of Sciences, the National Academy of Engineering, and the Institute of Medicine.

The National Academy of Sciences is a private, nonprofit, self-perpetuating society of distinguished scholars engaged in scientific and engineering research, dedicated to the furtherance of science and technology and to their use for the general welfare. Upon the authority of the charter granted to it by the Congress in 1863, the Academy has a mandate that requires it to advise the federal government on scientific and technical matters. Dr. Bruce M. Alberts is president of the National Academy of Sciences.

The National Academy of Engineering was established in 1964, under the charter of the National Academy of Sciences, as a parallel organization of outstanding engineers. It is autonomous in its administration and in the selection of its members, sharing with the National Academy of Sciences the responsibility for advising the federal government. The National Academy of Engineering also sponsors engineering programs aimed at meeting national needs, encourages education and research, and recognizes the superior achievements of engineers. Dr. William A. Wulf is interim president of the National Academy of Engineering.

The Institute of Medicine was established in 1970 by the National Academy of Sciences to secure the services of eminent members of appropriate professions in the examination of policy matters pertaining to the health of the public. The Institute acts under the responsibility given to the National Academy of Sciences by its congressional charter to be an adviser to the federal government and, upon its own initiative, to identify issues of medical care, research, and education. Dr. Kenneth I. Shine is president of the Institute of Medicine.

The National Research Council was organized by the National Academy of Sciences in 1916 to associate the broad community of science and technology with the Academy's purposes of furthering knowledge and advising the federal government. Functioning in accordance with general policies determined by the Academy, the Council has become the principal operating agency of both the National Academy of Sciences and the National Academy of Engineering in providing services to the government, the public, and the scientific and engineering communities. The Council is administered jointly by both Academies and the Institute of Medicine. Dr. Bruce M. Alberts and Dr. William A. Wulf are chairman and interim vice chairman, respectively, of the National Research Council.

This study was supported by the National Aeronautics and Space Administration under contract No. NASW-4938. Any opinions, findings, conclusions, or recommendations expressed in this publication are those of the author(s) and do not necessarily reflect the view of the organizations or agencies that provided support for the project.

Library of Congress Catalog Card Number 97-65884
International Standard Book Number 0-309-05688-8

Additional copies are available for sale from:

National Academy Press
Box 285
2101 Constitution Ave., N.W.
Washington, DC 20055
800-624-6242
202-334-3313 (in the Washington Metropolitan Area)
http://www.nap.edu

Printed in the United States of America

Committee on the Effects of Aircraft-Pilot Coupling on Flight Safety

DUANE T. McRUER (chair), Systems Technology, Inc.
CARL S. DROSTE, Lockheed Martin Tactical Aircraft Systems
R. JOHN HANSMAN, JR., Massachusetts Institute of Technology
RONALD A. HESS, University of California–Davis
DAVID P. LeMASTER, Wright Laboratory
STUART MATTHEWS, Flight Safety Foundation
JOHN D. McDONNELL, McDonnell Douglas Aerospace
JAMES McWHA, Boeing Commercial Airplane Group
WILLIAM W. MELVIN, Air Line Pilots Association; Delta Air Lines (retired)
RICHARD W. PEW, BBN Corporation

Staff

ALAN ANGLEMAN, Study Director
JOANN CLAYTON-TOWNSEND, Director, Aeronautics and Space Engineering Board
MARY MESZAROS, Senior Project Assistant

Aeronautics and Space Engineering Board Liaison

JOHN K. BUCKNER, Lockheed Martin Tactical Aircraft Systems (retired)

Technical Liaisons

RALPH A'HARRAH, National Aeronautics and Space Administration
JIM ASHLEY, Federal Aviation Administration
DAVID L. KEY, U.S. Army
TOM LAWRENCE, U.S. Navy

Preface

Unfavorable aircraft-pilot coupling (APC) events include a broad set of undesirable—and sometimes hazardous—phenomena that are associated with less-than-ideal interactions between pilots and aircraft. As civil and military aircraft technologies advance, pilot-aircraft interactions are becoming more complex. Recently, there have been accidents and incidents attributed to adverse APC in military aircraft. In addition, APC has been implicated in some civilian incidents. In response to this situation, and at the request of the National Aeronautics and Space Administration, the National Research Council established the Committee on the Effects of Aircraft-Pilot Coupling on Flight Safety. This committee evaluated the current state of knowledge about adverse APC and processes that may be used to eliminate it from military and commercial aircraft.

The committee analyzed the information it collected and developed a set of findings and recommendations for consideration by the U.S. Air Force, Navy, and Army; National Aeronautics and Space Administration; and Federal Aviation Administration. In particular, the committee concluded that in the short term the risk posed by adverse APC could be reduced by increased awareness of APC possibilities and more disciplined application of existing tools and capabilities throughout the development, test, and certification process. However, new approaches are also needed to address the APC risk faced by many advanced aircraft designs. In order to develop new approaches, long-term efforts are needed in the area of APC assessment criteria, analysis tools, and simulation capabilities. (See Chapter 7 for a complete list of the committee's findings and recommendations.)

The study committee met four times between September 1995 and June 1996. (See Appendix A for a list of committee members and their professional background.) To ensure that the committee's work included a broad range of perspectives, the second and third meetings included workshop presentations involving 38 outside individuals with experience in aircraft research, design, development, manufacture, test, and operations. The committee's outreach also extended internationally to France, Germany, Russia, Sweden, and the United Kingdom.

The committee wishes to thank all of its meeting participants, who are listed in Appendix B, for their contributions to the work of the committee. The committee also expresses special thanks for the assistance provided by each of its liaisons (see page *iii*).

Duane T. McRuer

DUANE T. McRUER
Committee Chair

Contents

Tables and Figures

TABLES

FIGURES

Executive Summary

Unfavorable aircraft-pilot coupling (APC) events are rare, unexpected, and unintended excursions in aircraft attitude and flight path caused by anomalous interactions between the aircraft and the pilot. The temporal pattern of these pilot-vehicle system (PVS) excursions can be oscillatory or divergent (non-oscillatory). The pilot's interactions with the aircraft can form either a closed-loop or open-loop system, depending on whether or not the pilot's responses are tightly coupled to the aircraft response. When the dynamics of the aircraft (including the flight control system [FCS]) and the dynamics of the pilot combine to produce an unstable PVS, the result is called an APC event.

Although it is often difficult to pinpoint the cause of specific APC events, a majority of severe APC events result from deficiencies in the design of the aircraft (especially with regard to the FCS) that result in adverse coupling of the pilot with the aircraft. In certain circumstances, this adverse coupling produces unintended oscillations or divergences when the pilot attempts to precisely maneuver the aircraft. If the PVS instability takes the form of an oscillation, the APC event is called a "pilot-involved oscillation" (PIO). PIOs differ from aircraft oscillations caused by deliberate, pilot-imposed periodic control motions, such as "stick-pumping," that are open-loop in character. An open-loop, forced oscillation does not constitute a PIO. If the unstable motions of the closed-loop PVS are divergent rather than oscillatory in nature, they are referred to as either APC events or as non-oscillatory APC events.

APC events can result if the pilot is operating with a behavioral mode that is inappropriate for the task at hand, and such events are properly ascribed to pilot error. However, the committee believes that most severe APC events attributed to pilot error are the result of adverse APC that misleads the pilot into taking actions that contribute to the severity of the event. It is often possible, after the fact, to carefully analyze an event and identify a sequence of actions that the pilot could have taken to overcome the aircraft design deficiencies. However, it is typically not feasible for the pilot to identify and execute the required actions in real time.

PIO phenomena comprise a complete spectrum. At one end of the spectrum is a momentary, easily corrected, low-amplitude bobble, a type of oscillation often encountered by pilots getting used to new configurations—basically a learning experience. This type of oscillation can happen on any aircraft and has been experienced by most pilots at one time or another. At the other end of the spectrum is a fully-developed, large amplitude PIO, a chilling and terrifying event that jeopardizes the safety of the aircraft, crew, and passengers. Fortunately, severe PIOs are rare.

Other severe APC events have been noted in which the excursions in aircraft motion diverge over time rather than oscillate. The few events of this nature that have been positively identified have had serious consequences. Large amplitude, dangerous PIOs and non-oscillatory APC events are the particular concerns of this report.

Recently, there have been several highly visible APC-related accidents involving military aircraft, as well as a number of incidents involving civil aircraft. At the same time, there has been widespread introduction of new fly-by-wire (FBW) FCSs into commercial transports. Almost all new FBW-equipped aircraft have exhibited APC events at some time during development, and these untoward coincidences have captured the attention of policymakers, test pilots, technical managers, and engineers. Although FBW systems are not inherently more or less susceptible to severe APC events, the flurry of incidents in aircraft development programs suggests that some side effects have not been fully explored or anticipated. Thus, as a matter of prudence the National Aeronautics and Space Administration asked the Aeronautics and Space Engineering Board of the National Research Council to conduct a study to assess APC-related aspects of recent incidents and accidents, aircraft development processes, the introduction of FBW and fly-by-light technology into FCSs, and national and international efforts devoted to APC research. This report is the result of that study, and it recommends steps that could be taken to improve aviation safety by reducing the kinds of APC problems seen recently and countering new types of APC problems that may arise.

The following high-level conclusions of the study committee are worth highlighting. (Subsequent sections include the committee's key findings and recommendations, and all findings and recommendations are listed in Chapter 7.)

- There are many varieties of oscillatory and non-oscillatory APC events. Although none of these is welcome, only a rare subset is dangerous. Among the dangerous ones are events that exhibit "cliff-like" characteristics, which means that a PVS may fly superbly up to the sudden onset of a dramatic and potentially catastrophic APC event. What these severe APCs are, when they are likely to occur, and how to find (and fix) them are key issues.

- Most of the severe PIOs for which flight recordings exist have exhibited oscillations characterized by rate limited responses in control surface actuators or effectors. (Control surface actuators and effectors are rate or position limited when commanded movement exceeds limits imposed by design intent or physical structure on the rate of movement or extreme position of the control surface.) In most cases the pilots indicated that the onset of the PIO was sudden, unexpected, and cliff-like.
- Piloted simulations have proved to be useful for investigating APC tendencies. However, neither piloted simulations nor available design and testing criteria can guarantee that a new aircraft will not be involved in an APC event.
- Severe APC events are invariably new "discoveries" that often occur in transient and highly unusual circumstances. To avoid their discovery by operational pilots under unfavorable circumstances, test pilots must be allowed some freedom to search for APC tendencies in simulations and flight tests.
- Data on recent APC events indicate that they are not uncommon in development testing where data recording and pilot reports are sufficient for causes to be determined and solutions developed. There are only a few reports of severe APC events in operational aircraft, but because there are no mandatory reporting requirements and recordings are often inadequate, the danger cannot be assessed adequately.
- The committee was disturbed by the lack of awareness of severe APC events among pilots, engineers, regulatory authorities, and accident investigators.

THE AIRCRAFT-PILOT COUPLING EXPERIENCE

APC events usually occur when the pilot is engaged in a highly demanding, closed-loop control task. For example, many of the reported APC events have taken place during air-to-air refueling operations or approaches and landings, especially if the pilot is concerned about low fuel, adverse weather, emergencies, or other circumstances. Under these conditions, the pilot's involvement in closed-loop control is intense, and rapid response and precise performance of the PVS are necessary. Even so, these operations usually occur routinely without APC problems. APC events do not occur unless there is a transient triggering event that interrupts the already highly-demanding PVS operations or requires an even higher level of precision. Typical triggers include shifts in the dynamics of the effective aircraft (the combination of the aircraft and FCS) caused by increases in the amplitude of pilot commands, FCS changes, minor mechanical malfunctions, or severe atmospheric disturbances. Other triggers can stem from mismatches between the pilot's expectations and reality.

PIOs have been part of aviation history since the beginning of manned flight, and severe PIOs persist in spite of major efforts to eliminate them. When one kind of PIO occurs, usually unexpectedly, it stirs corrective actions. The experience is generally useful, in that the conditions thought to underlie that type of PIO tend to be avoided in designing new aircraft. As other PIOs occur under different circumstances, the cycle is repeated. With time, understanding improves and some causes are circumvented, but the occurrence of closed-loop oscillations remains a constant; only the details change with the aircraft and FCS technology.

From the pilot's perspective, there are three varieties of PIO experiences, ranging from benign learning experiences to severe and potentially dangerous oscillations. The benign "bobbles" are easily countered by the pilot's exit from the closed-loop PVS. By contrast, in many severe PIOs the pilot becomes locked into behavior that sustains the oscillation, even though the pilot often feels totally disconnected from the system. If the deficiencies in effective aircraft dynamics are essentially linear in nature, such as excessive time lag in response to a pilot input, a Category I PIO may result. If the effective aircraft dynamics change as a function of pilot-command amplitude or of FCS mode shifts, thereby creating a nonlinear sudden-onset change (a "cliff") in the effective aircraft dynamics, the resulting PIO is assigned either to Category II (when the dominant nonlinearities are associated with rate or position limiting of the control surfaces) or Category III (when the nonlinear changes are more complex). The Category II and III PIOs are particularly insidious because the effective aircraft dynamics and the associated flying qualities can be good right up to the instant the PIO begins. Identifying the potential for these PIOs, which almost always occur under unusual conditions when the PVS is operating near the margins, is a major challenge to test pilots and engineers. An extensive search process with a "discovery" mentality is needed to ensure that Category II or III tendencies are not overlooked.

Non-oscillatory APC events are not as well defined or understood as PIOs. Even if the pilot is extremely active and initiates many control reversals, the aircraft does not necessarily respond in an oscillatory fashion. Instead, a buildup of lags in the response of the aircraft's control effectors to the pilot's commands may ultimately lead to a divergence from the intended aircraft movement. As in the case of severe PIOs, pilots in these cases often report a sense of feeling detached from the aircraft behavior in terms of both awareness of what is happening and in terms of the temporal connections between pilot command and aircraft response.

Finding. Adverse APC events are rare, unintended, and unexpected oscillations or divergences of the pilot-aircraft system. APC events are fundamentally interactive and occur during highly demanding tasks when environmental, pilot, or aircraft dynamic changes create or trigger mismatches between actual and expected aircraft responses.

IMPACT OF NEW TECHNOLOGY

As phenomena in aviation history, APC problems have often been associated with the introduction of new technologies, functionalities, or complexities. There is a time lapse before flight experience with a new technology reveals the subtle changes in effective aircraft dynamics that may increase the susceptibility of a new aircraft to APC events. This partly explains why APC problems are more prevalent in military aircraft, which have traditionally introduced advanced technologies, and less common in civil aircraft, which have tended to adopt new technologies only after they have been proven in military aircraft. The prevalence of APC problems in military rather than commercial aircraft may also be associated with the nature of military operations, which frequently include maneuvers that require higher pilot gains than are commonly used on commercial aircraft.

FBW technology, which for this report includes fly-by-light technology, is a recent example of a new technology that has migrated from military to civil aircraft. The application of FBW technology has created FCSs that confer important overall system advantages in terms of performance, weight reduction, stability and control, operational flexibility, and maintenance requirements. FBW also offers opportunities for novel approaches to solving all kinds of problems with aircraft stability and control (including correcting APC tendencies). Yet, the flexibility inherent in FBW technology has the potential for creating unwanted new side effects and unanticipated problems.

In an aircraft equipped with a FBW FCS, information is transmitted from the cockpit to the control surfaces entirely by electrical means. The cockpit control device may not indicate to the pilot when the control surfaces are rate or position limited. The result may be a mismatch between the pilot's expectations and the aircraft's actual response, which can directly contribute to an APC event. In addition, FBW technology allows aircraft designers to design an FCS that features an elaborate set of system modes intended to enhance aircraft performance for a variety of missions under all expected flight conditions. When properly implemented, shifts between these system modes are smooth and unobtrusive and do not interfere with the pilot's operation of the aircraft. However, the complexity inherent in an advanced multiredundant FBW FCS makes it difficult for the designers, much less the pilots, to anticipate all of the possible interactions between the FCS and the pilot. The

FCS may operate in ways that the pilot does not expect and does not recognize, thereby increasing the potential of encountering an APC event. As the potential for untoward events expands with the introduction of new technologies, increased vigilance is necessary to ensure that new systems do not inadvertently increase the susceptibility of new aircraft to APC events.

Finding. APC problems are often associated with the introduction of new designs, technologies, functions, or complexities. New technologies, such as FBW and fly-by-light flight control systems, are constantly being incorporated into aircraft. As a result, opportunities for APC are likely to persist or even increase, and greater vigilance is necessary to ensure that new technologies do not inadvertently increase the susceptibility of new aircraft to APC events.

AIRCRAFT-PILOT COUPLING EVENTS AS A CURRENT PROBLEM IN AVIATION

A major task of the committee was to assess the current status of APC events as a safety problem in aviation. In the context of aircraft development and testing, the record clearly shows that although adverse APC events are rare, they can pose a major safety concern. The same record also provides an extraordinary set of recent examples that should alert project and engineering managers, design engineers, test pilots, and aircraft operators to the need to address concerns about APC events as a central flying qualities and safety issue. These concerns can be addressed through detailed test plans, elaborate flight-test data recorders, and highly trained pilots like the ones who participate in the developmental stages of new aviation technology. Addressing these concerns will ensure that APC events that occur during development become matters of record.

When an aircraft enters operational service, the elaborate flight data recorders are routinely removed. The flight data recorders that are installed on many commercial aircraft employ a limited number of channels and sample rates; many military aircraft have no flight data recorders at all. For these and other reasons, confirmed APC-related incidents or accidents on operational FBW aircraft are quite rare.

The occurrence of PIOs or other APC events at some point in the development of almost all FBW aircraft, contrasted with the almost total absence of APC events reported in operational stages, is viewed by the committee as a "curious disconnect." The hope is that all major APC tendencies have been discovered and corrected in the course of development, but because of the limited recording and reporting procedures in operations, this cannot be confirmed. Consequently, the committee was not able to assess fully the exposure of operational fleets to APC events.

Finding. APC problems have occurred more often in military and experimental aircraft, which have traditionally introduced advanced technologies, than in civil aircraft.

Finding. Recently, civil and military transport FBW aircraft have experienced APC problems during development and testing, and some APC events have occurred in recent commercial aircraft service, although they may not always have been recognized as such.

INCREASING AWARENESS

The committee has observed that APC events are perceived by the majority of the aviation community as exotic happenings that are occasionally documented by spectacular video footage shown on the evening news but are not of major concern. This complacent attitude is reinforced by a lack of awareness, understanding, and relevant experience. This shortcoming should be addressed through improved education and training of personnel involved in aircraft design, simulation, testing, certification, operations, and accident investigation.

A dramatic way to enhance awareness is to expose flight test pilots and engineers to actual APC events in flight and thereby indelibly imprint on them the insidious character and the danger of such phenomena. Although this could be done at relatively little expense using existing variable stability aircraft, this kind of training for test pilots and engineers is not common in industry, the Federal Aviation Administration, or the Department of Defense. (It may also be possible to use ground-based simulators for APC awareness training, especially for Category I APC events, but they are not likely to make the same sort of dramatic impression on pilots as in-flight experiences.) The committee believes test pilots need specialized training to improve their ability to detect adverse APC characteristics. Test pilots tend to adapt very quickly to new aircraft, and they may unconsciously compensate for deficiencies in a FCS that, in some circumstances, could contribute to an APC event. Therefore, their training should also include aggressive searches for tendencies that could lead to APC events.

Because most line pilots have not been trained to recognize and report adverse APC characteristics, they often attribute PIOs to deficiencies in their flying skills. The committee suspects that this tends to limit reporting of adverse APC events to safety reporting systems.

Appropriate training is equally important for accident investigators and others involved in evaluating flight operations. Investigators should be knowledgeable about APC hazards and how to identify them. The improving capabilities of flight data recording systems will aid investigators in determining whether APC phenomena contributed to specific incidents and accidents.

Recommendation. Insufficient attention to APC phenomena generally seems to be associated with a lack of understanding and relevant experience; this shortcoming should be addressed through improved education about APC phenomena for pilots and other personnel involved in aircraft design, simulation, testing, certification, operation, and accident investigation.

ELIMINATING AIRCRAFT-PILOT COUPLING EVENTS

To increase the likelihood of finding major APC tendencies during the development process, the committee recommends that a disciplined and structured approach be taken in the design, development, testing, and certification of aircraft. This approach is intended to improve existing techniques for mitigating the risk of adverse APC and to expedite the adoption of new techniques as they become available.

Management

The elimination of APC events requires both an effective technical approach and a highly supportive management structure. In the past, a possible susceptibility to APC was sometimes detected during simulations and analysis early in the development of new aircraft but was dismissed by managers or designers as premature or irrelevant because the susceptibility was associated with tasks that were viewed as uncharacteristic of actual flight operations. In other cases, APC susceptibility has been inadvertently introduced into new aircraft with design changes that were not fully assessed for their impact on APC characteristics. Program managers and designers should implement a highly structured systems-engineering approach that involves all relevant disciplines in the APC-elimination process from early in the program through entry into service.

Design Criteria

Good "flying qualities" are fundamental to the elimination of adverse APC. The starting point for military aircraft is compliance with the requirements in MIL-STD-1797A and Draft MIL-STD-1797A Update.[70,71] Compliance lessens APC tendencies in classical fixed-wing aircraft with modest stability augmentation systems and conventional fully-powered surface actuating systems. Rotorcraft that meet the requirements of ADS-33D[68] are also likely to be more resistant to APC events. However, these specifications, like the criteria upon which they are based, do not adequately address the susceptibility of aircraft to Category II and III PIOs and to non-oscillatory APCs. These requirements should be supplemented early in the design process by appropriate criteria and metrics selected and tailored, as necessary, to guide development teams in assessing the flying qualities and susceptibility of new aircraft to adverse APC. The APC criteria should emphasize highly demanding, closed-loop operations of the PVS, as well as precision maneuvering characteristics. The criteria should be viewed as a means of alerting the analysis and design teams to features that can increase the risk of APC. Current design criteria cannot guarantee that a given design will be free of adverse APC characteristics in flight. Appropriate combinations of available APC criteria are generally useful for assessing the susceptibility of aircraft designs to most types of linear, oscillatory APC events (i.e., Category I PIOs). Available criteria do not effectively address more complex types of APC events—Category II and III PIOs and non-oscillatory APC events. Research on APC design assessment criteria should focus on these less understood types of APC events; a coordinated approach that combines experiments with the development of new analysis approaches is essential.

Simulation and Flight Tests

Ground and in-flight simulators and pilots who are sensitive to APC tendencies can contribute to the development of a FCS with satisfactory APC characteristics. The potential of simulators to reproduce APC events that have been encountered in flight has been repeatedly demonstrated. However, the continuing occurrence of unexpected APC events in flight also illustrates the limited effectiveness of current simulation technologies and procedures for predicting APC events. Existing simulation and analysis tools should be refined to be more specific, selective, and accurate predictors. A high priority should be placed on research to develop predictive simulation protocols and tasks and to validate simulation test results with flight tests.

Fixed-base simulators may not always reveal the existence of adverse APC tendencies because of (1) the lack of acceleration cues; (2) less-than-satisfactory visual systems; (3) inadequate simulation of major FCS details, especially inceptors and FCS characteristics that come into play when PVS operations are at or near transitions or other conditions that define margins; and (4) the difficulty of instilling stress and a sense of urgency in the pilot. Moving-base simulators may be more effective than fixed-base simulators in some parts of the flight envelope, although they too can have the deficiencies listed above, as well as the oddities of motion washout and other artifacts. The committee believes that a high-quality visual display is more effective than a moving base because most simulations involve instrument-rated pilots who are trained to rely upon visual rather than acceleration cues.

In-flight simulation solves many of the problems inherent in ground simulation if the effective aircraft dynamics, including inceptors, are well simulated. In-flight simulation can be especially valuable for increasing the APC awareness of test and operational pilots and flight test engineers and for demonstrating and conducting research on cliff-like APC phenomena (Category II and III PIOs and non-oscillatory APCs). Highly focused flight-test evaluations of prototypes or pre-certification aircraft can be particularly helpful for identifying flight situations that might be susceptible to APC, as well as for providing the final measures of performance.

Throughout the simulation and flight test process, pilots must be assigned appropriate tasks (see Chapter 4) in order to evaluate APC characteristics effectively. Because APC events are commonly associated with highly demanding, precisely controlled aircraft movements, simulation and flight tests used for assessing APC tendencies should include such tasks as aggressive acquisition maneuvers, aggressive tracking maneuvers, mode transitions, formation flying and aerial refueling, approach and landing, and special tracking tasks.

It is important that a variety of repeatable tasks be included to ensure that APC assessments are comprehensive and verifiable. In addition, many pilots should be involved in simulation and flight tests to ensure that the aircraft will accommodate a wide range of piloting skills; two or three test pilots are not enough to conduct a thorough evaluation and examination if APC characteristics are marginally acceptable. An aggressive search for APC tendencies is especially important in flight regimes where cliff-like phenomena are most likely to appear.

Recommendation. A disciplined and structured approach should be taken in the design, development, testing, and certification stages to maximize the effectiveness of existing techniques for mitigating the risk of adverse APC tendencies and for expediting the incorporation of new techniques as they become available. This is especially important in areas where effective procedures and standards do not currently exist (e.g., FAA certification standards).

INTERIM PRESCRIPTION FOR AVOIDING SEVERE AIRCRAFT-PILOT COUPLING EVENTS

This report stresses the need for enhanced awareness of APC phenomena and an orderly and structured design and development process to address this problem. Although no definitive criteria are applicable to all types of APC events, the technical guidelines that appear below can confer immunity to most severe APC events. The committee recognizes that readers concerned with specifics may find the following discussion of processes and criteria too general, even as other readers who are unfamiliar with APC phenomenology may find the details of some technical descriptions difficult to understand.

Reduce Category I Pilot-Induced Oscillation Tendencies

Implications for Design of the Effective Aircraft Dynamics

Reduce time lags in the high-frequency effective aircraft dynamics. To reduce tendencies for attitude-dominant PIOs, increase the frequency range over which a pilot hypothetically operating in a pure-gain (proportional control) mode can exert closed-loop control on aircraft attitude. Counter possible interactions between the pilot and higher-frequency modes of the effective aircraft dynamics.

Suitable Metrics and Criteria

Ensure that inceptor characteristics, flexible modes of the aircraft structure, and other elements of a PVS that incorporates a pure-gain pilot do not create high frequency closed-loop resonances. Three criteria (i.e., the Gain/Phase Template Plus ω_{180} /Average Phase Rate criterion, the Dropback criterion, and the Aircraft-Bandwidth/Phase Delay criterion) can provide useful warnings and design guidance.

Minimize Category II and III Pilot-Induced Oscillation Tendencies

Implications for Design of the Effective Aircraft Dynamics

Provide seamless transitions when the FCS switches between control modes or control laws. Minimize transitions that create large increases in the phase lag or gain that the FCS applies to the pilot's commands, especially simultaneous increases in both.

Suitable Metrics and Criteria

Develop metrics and criteria for predicting Category II and III PIO tendencies. (Currently, such criteria do not exist.) Reduce the effects of phase lag introduced by rate limiting by providing liberal rate limits and minimizing the need for large pilot commands during critical closed-loop tasks. Command-gain changes and pre- to post-transition dynamic shifts of no more than about 3 dB (50 percent) are tentative lower limits for tasks that require the pilot to exert tight closed-loop control.

Examine the Possibility of Non-Oscillatory Aircraft-Pilot Coupling Events

In searching for unexpected non-oscillatory APC events, consider special maneuvers, pilot commands, and FCS inputs that may effectively increase the time lag between the pilot's command and its reflection at the control surface.

Conduct Assessments and Evaluations Using Simulators

Implications for Design

Provide simulator characteristics that are valid reflections of effective aircraft dynamics, especially for high PVS frequencies and conditions where FCS operations are nonlinear. Extensively examine situations that analysis has indicated are marginal with respect to the occurrence of Category I APC events. Conduct a specialized and detailed search for potentially critical Category II and III (cliff-like) situations using an impartial team of experienced FCS engineers. Include circumstances that may require large pilot inputs, high pilot gain, or FCS shifts between modes and/or control laws.

Implications for Test Execution

Use test input sequences that put maximal stress on the PVS. Include periods of active, freelance pilot operations to search for potential limiting conditions (see Table 4-2). Also include a broad spectrum of test pilots and operational pilots. Examine maneuvers and command sequences that may effectively increase the time lag between the pilot's command and the control surface effector's reflection of this command.

Conduct Flight Evaluations

Use flight evaluations, which are closely related to simulation tests, to build on the results of simulation. In particular, use test input sequences that stress the PVS to extremes and include a spectrum of pilots. Conduct tests of situations where PVS performance was previously determined or suspected to be marginal, as well as conditions that have no parallel in simulation (e.g., situations that involve very high frequency modes or acceleration-sensitive phenomena). Devote an investigatory phase, with appropriate safety measures, to an active and aggressive search by pilots for potential, cliff-like PIO conditions, such as conditions involving rate or position limits. Include carefree freelance operations that provide test pilots with "open time" to experiment freely.

ALTERNATIVE APPROACHES

The approaches used to address APC risk in the U.S. and international civil and military aviation communities are not consistent. Some organizations rely heavily on the analysis of new designs in accordance with formal APC criteria. Others rely primarily on empirical methods and rules of thumb based on experience with prior aircraft. The committee did not find any approach that consistently produces aircraft free of adverse APC characteristics. APC events thus remain a threat, and the potential for tragedy will persist until the goal of reducing APC risk is aggressively pursued.

Manufacturers of civil and military aircraft often consider the approaches they use to reduce the risk of adverse APC as a component of their proprietary design and manufacturing process. In addition, the APC characteristics of current aircraft are often treated as proprietary or classified performance data. These attitudes tend to inhibit the exchange of APC-related information and interfere with cooperative efforts to reduce the risk. Nevertheless, the committee believes that, in the interest of aviation safety, the free exchange of APC-related information on design and manufacturing processes and on aircraft performance characteristics should be encouraged throughout the military and civil aviation communities, nationally and internationally. This report, which contains a great deal of data, information, and procedures that would normally be considered proprietary, is a step in this direction.

1

Aircraft-Pilot Coupling Problems: Definitions, Descriptions, and History

INTRODUCTION

"Aircraft-pilot coupling (APC) events" are inadvertent, unwanted aircraft attitude and flight path motions that originate in anomalous interactions between the aircraft and the pilot. The concept of the pilot and aircraft as constituents of a "pilot-vehicle system" (PVS) is central to understanding APC events. Historically, the most common APC events have been sustained, oscillatory motions of the PVS. These motions include changes in the aircraft attitude and flight path caused by the flight control system (FCS) and generally associated with pilot inputs. Oscillatory APC events have historically been referred to as "pilot-induced oscillations" (PIOs).

The committee has adopted APC phraseology for two reasons. The first is to remove the presumption of blame implicit in the term "pilot-induced"; although it is often difficult to pinpoint the cause of specific APC events, a majority of severe APC events result from deficiencies in the design of the aircraft (especially with regard to the FCS) that result in adverse coupling of the pilot with the aircraft. The second reason for referring to APC events instead of PIOs is to expand the focus of the term to include other extreme, unwanted PVS motions that, although not necessarily oscillatory, still derive from inadvertent pilot-vehicle interactions. An excellent, well documented example of a non-oscillatory APC event is the second JAS 39 accident, which is listed in Table 1-2 and described in Chapter 2 (at the end of the Non-Oscillatory Aircraft-Pilot Coupling section).

Both oscillatory and non-oscillatory APC events represent a fundamental discord between the pilot's intentions and the aircraft's response. Properties of the aircraft are contributing factors to the adverse motions. APC events are collaborations between the pilot and the aircraft in that they occur only when the pilot attempts to control what the aircraft does. Indeed, the effective aircraft, left to the control of the FCS, will ordinarily remain dynamically stable in flight. For this reason, pilot error is often listed as the cause of accidents and incidents that include an APC event. However, the committee believes that most severe APC events attributed to pilot error are the result of adverse APC that misleads the pilot into taking actions that contribute to the severity of the event. In these situations, it is often possible, after the fact, to analyze the event carefully and identify a sequence of actions that the pilot could have taken to overcome the aircraft design deficiencies and avoid the event. However, it is typically not feasible for the pilot to identify and execute the required actions in real time.

Because the pilot's actions depend, in part, on the motions of the aircraft in response to pilot commands, the aircraft and pilot dynamics form a closed-loop feedback control system.* The pilot is said to be "operating closed-loop" or to be "in the loop." Adverse APC characteristics can therefore be identified as instabilities in a closed-loop feedback control system. Oscillatory APC events have been the easiest to identify and comprehend and have therefore received the most attention in this study (as they have in the past). These PVS oscillations will be referred to hereafter as "pilot-involved oscillations" (PIOs) without thereby ascribing blame.

Non-oscillatory APC events, such as divergences,* are less well defined because the aircraft motions can be far more diverse and the cause-effect relationships more difficult to comprehend. Nonetheless, new possibilities for APC have arisen with the use of multifunction, special purpose control surfaces and subsystems intended to enhance performance and stability and control, and with the advent of fly-by-wire (FBW)* FCS technology that makes many new system concepts and improvements feasible. Foremost, but not alone, among these new possibilities is the spatial (mechanical) disconnect—with consequent temporal separations (typically tenths of a second)—between the pilot's command actions and the aircraft control effectors' reflection of the pilot's intent. With FBW controls, the pilot does not receive a direct indication through the cockpit control device when a control-surface actuator is rate limited,* whereas with some older direct hydraulic controls, mechanical resistance to further command movement indicates that the actuator is rate limited. Similarly, FBW controls do not give direct indications of rate limitations included in the software.

When stability augmentation systems (SASs)* and other FCS-associated subsystems share control effectors with direct pilot inputs, the pilot's authority over the control surfaces can also be substantially reduced. The pilot, unaware

---

*Terms marked by an asterisk are defined in the glossary.

that the systems are operating at their limits, may call for a greater response from the control surface than is allowed by the system's rate or position limits* for that effector. The resulting "disharmony" between the pilot's intentions and the aircraft's response can significantly affect the pilot's comprehension of the overall status of the PVS. All of these effects may be present and quantifiable in oscillatory PVS behavior, but for non-oscillatory interactions they are more of a potential problem because they may not be positively identified or exemplified. Consequently, this report focuses more on system oscillations than on potential, non-oscillatory interactions.

Initial Concrete Example

PIOs have been around since the time of the Wright brothers, giving them an unambiguous seniority among flying qualities* problems.[42] In terms of severity and consequences, pilot-vehicle oscillatory phenomena comprise a complete spectrum. The oscillations may be of the temporary, easily corrected, low-amplitude variety often encountered by pilots when getting the feel of a new configuration—basically a learning experience. These oscillations can happen on any aircraft and have been experienced by most pilots at one time or another. On the other hand, a fully developed, large-amplitude oscillation with near or actual catastrophic consequences is a terrifying event that jeopardizes the safety of the aircraft, passengers, and crew. Severe PIOs are either difficult or impossible for the pilot to arrest.

The in-flight recording of Figure 1-1 illustrates a severe PIO and should motivate interest in this phenomenon. This event occurred with an early version of the T-38 trainer, and it remains a historical landmark for several reasons: the aircraft was equipped with instruments to collect detailed flight data; the incident was about as severe as one can get without an actual breakup of the aircraft; and the event has been extensively studied. As a result, this event has provided valuable insight into severe PIOs.

The time traces shown in Figure 1-1 indicate that the event was preceded by a low-amplitude, high-frequency oscillation involving only the pitch axis of the aircraft and the SAS; note that the force the pilot applied to the stick was zero during this pre-PIO phase. In other words, the initial oscillation was an instability of the SAS-aircraft combination with no pilot involvement. To eliminate the oscillation, the pilot disengaged the pitch SAS and entered the control loop in an attempt to counter the resulting upset.* Triggered by these events, at the pilot's intervention, a 1.2 Hz (7.4 rad/sec) oscillation developed very rapidly. In just a cycle or so, the oscillation had achieved an amplitude of ±5 g, increasing gradually to ±8 g, perilously near aircraft design limits. Recovery occurred when the pilot removed himself from the control loop. This example is given here to capture the reader's attention and to show that such events, although extremely unusual, can be very serious.

Although severe APC events are rare, they continue to occur, and, what is of more concern, they seem to be increasing in variety and complexity as aircraft systems advance. Large amplitude, potentially catastrophic, severe APCs can appear in many guises and can involve many factors. To understand these factors and their interactions, the PVS must be dissected in detail. Understanding the possibilities as well as the past examples involves a process of identifying, describing, and examining the constituents of severe APC problems and how they interact. This process begins with a description of the PVS, followed by a brief historical perspective.

PILOT-VEHICLE CLOSED-LOOP SYSTEM

The general physical structure of a PVS subject to one command input from the pilot is summarized in Figure 1-2. From the pilot's perspective, this is a "single-axis" situation in that the pilot's command is expressed by a single manipulation of a control inceptor. "Inceptor" is a catchall term for the pilot's control devices, such as the control stick or wheel for lateral control, the stick or column for longitudinal control, handles for controlling throttles and flaps, and pedals for controlling rudders. An inceptor may affect several vehicle control effectors (e.g., control surfaces)—for example, coordinated motions of aileron and rudder originated by a lateral stick deflection. This single-axis structure may encompass various inputs to the pilot. (The dynamics of the human pilot as an element within the closed-loop PVS can take several forms depending on the details of the specific system. A short description of these forms appears in Chapter 5 [see the section, Different Modes of Pilot Behavior]. A more extensive explanation is provided by McRuer.[42]) Examples of input to the pilot are: simple visual cues, such as pitch attitude; motion cues, such as normal acceleration at the pilot's location; composite signals, such as flight director error displays; or combinations of these inputs.

As shown in Figure 1-2, the inanimate elements of the system comprise the aircraft, FCS, and "displays." In principle, "displays" include all sources of sensory information the pilot uses to understand aircraft motion, especially those that derive from visual, motion-related, and aural modalities. The displays therefore include outside visual cues as well as cockpit instruments, proprioceptive* (e.g., perceived limb force and movement) inputs from inceptors, etc. In Figure 1-2, accelerations and angular velocities are shown as direct feedbacks to the pilot and as inputs to the display complex. Even aural signals from warning devices can contribute to the grand overall "display" that provides cues to the pilot. Because severe PIOs are almost always relatively high-frequency oscillations (0.2 to 3 Hz), only the "displayed" inputs that provide cues for the higher-frequency PVS loops are of practical consequence. This simplifies the analysis considerably and emphasizes as key cues the aircraft attitudes and accelerations and the pilot-perceived control forces and displacements (proprioceptive variables) at the inceptor level.

To represent the cues relevant to PIO, Figure 1-2 defines two slightly different entities that interact with the pilot. The first is the "effective aircraft dynamics," which consists of the aircraft as modified by the FCS. The second is the total dynamic entity with which the pilot interacts, the "controlled element," which includes certain elements of the display complex that contribute to the cue dynamics and are associated with the effective aircraft dynamics. In most APC events, the display complex quantities of interest include pitch or roll attitudes, which are visually perceived from the pilot's external field of view. In these cases, no distinction between the effective aircraft dynamics and the controlled element is necessary.

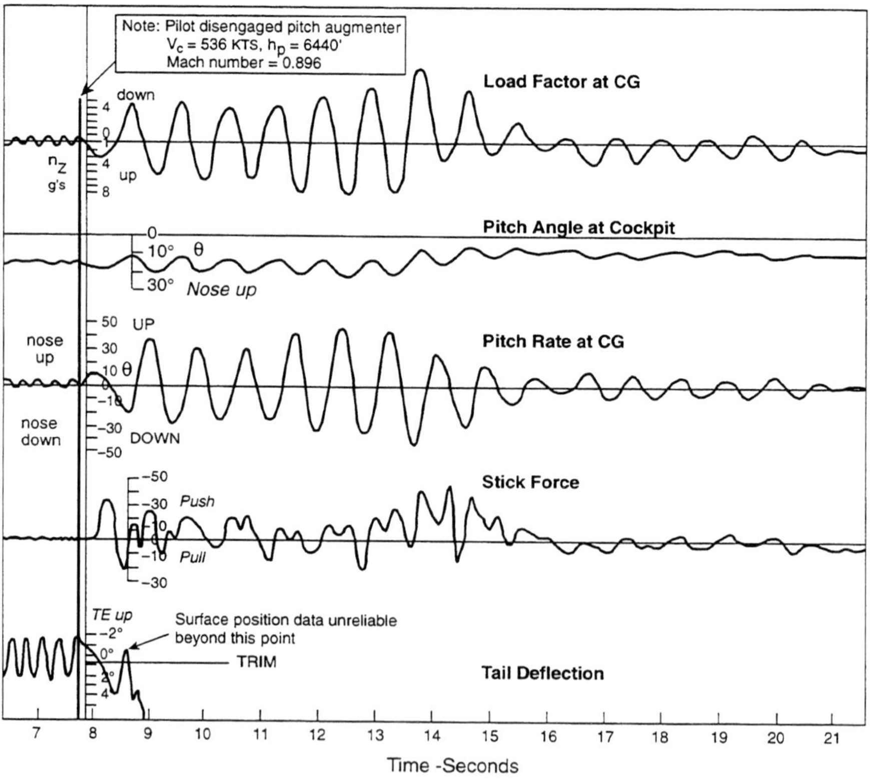

FIGURE 1-1 Flight recording of T-38 PIO. Adapted from: Ashkenas et al.[3]

NECESSARY CONDITIONS FOR OSCILLATORY AIRCRAFT-PILOT COUPLING EVENTS

The pilot, controlled element, task, and goal elements shown in Figure 1-2 are the principal constituents that can interact to cause a PIO when the PVS is a tightly-coupled closed-loop. Figure 1-3 shows the sufficient conditions for a continuous oscillation of the pilot–controlled-element system. These conditions can be satisfied only when the closed-loop PVS is operated with high pilot gain.*

Most flying tasks are accomplished with highly skilled discrete commands that are tailored for specific maneuvers and applied as open-loop inputs. Very few tracking-like operations demand full attention, continuous, closed-loop, pilot-controlled actions. Figure 1-3 lists some of the flight control tasks in which a high pilot gain is required to achieve necessary levels of closed-loop system dynamic performance and precision of control. Although they are a small subset of flight control tasks, most of them are well defined, ordinary, light operations.

By contrast, severe PIOs are extraordinary passages across stability boundaries. Although PIOs may, on occasion, appear to result from overly aggressive actions, they are more often associated with anomalous *changes* either in the pilot's behavior, the effective aircraft dynamics, or the display complex. These anomalies (the last item in Figure 1-3, Demanding or Unexpected Transitions) include conditions that induce or require one of the following responses:

- sudden major overall changes in the PVS configuration, such as wave off, target maneuvering, shift in goals, manual takeover, etc.
- modifications of the effective vehicle configuration (e.g., sudden changes in effective aircraft dynamics, such as FCS mode switching, autopilot disconnects when the aircraft is out of trim, or reconfigurations of control or power during go-arounds and aborts; low-altitude cargo extractions; afterburner light-offs; engine unstart; asymmetric stores release; SAS failures; maneuvering into Mach buffet;* or any changes in effective aircraft dynamics that are sensitive to pilot gain or driven by a shift in pilot action from small to large amplitude inputs)
- changes in the pilot's dynamics and/or the pilot-defined system architecture (e.g., shifts of dominant cues or pilot behavioral mode)

The unexpected and unusual nature of most severe oscillatory APC events implies an unusual precursor or "trigger" event. The fundamental characteristic of a trigger event is a mismatch between the pilot's control strategy and the effective aircraft dynamics that are being controlled. Triggers can arise either from external or internal sources. They may be major upsets,

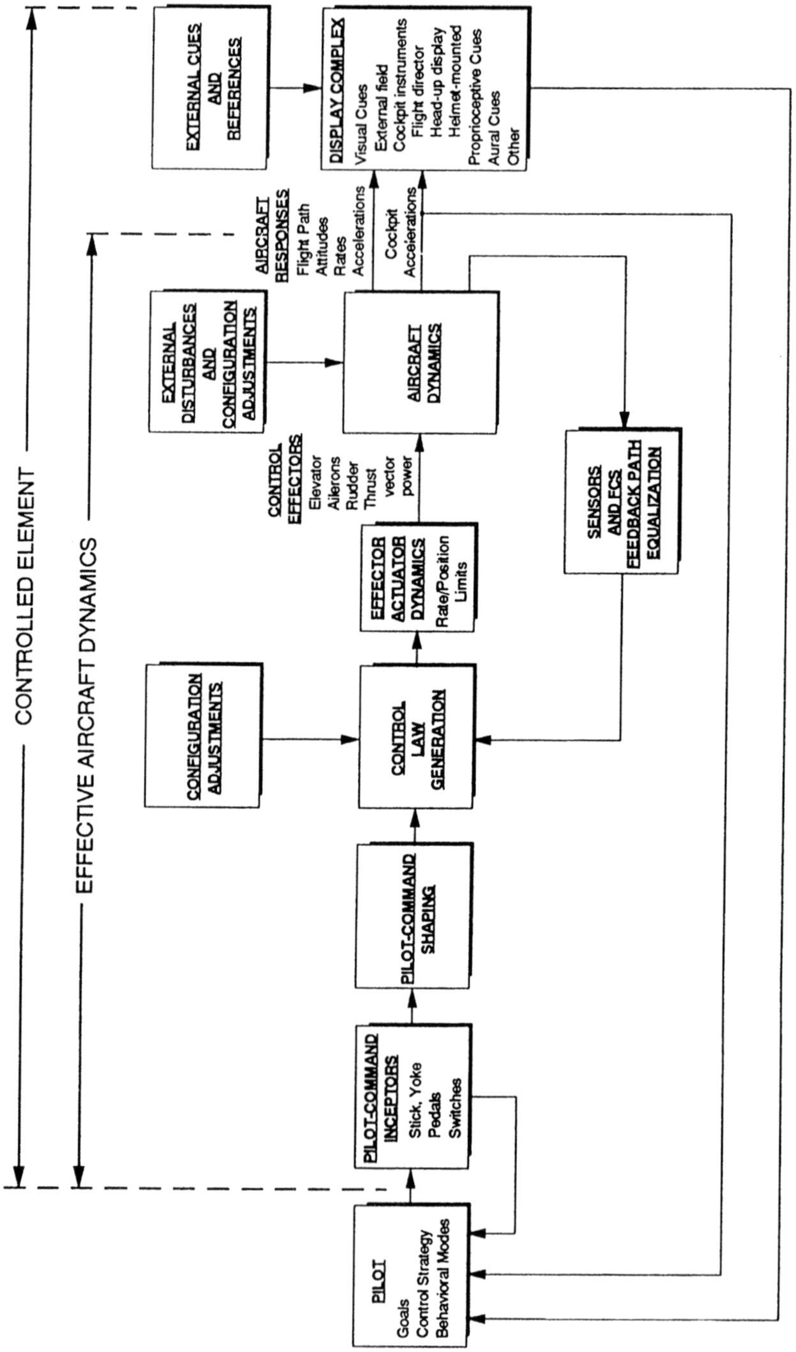

FIGURE 1-2 The pilot controlled-element system.

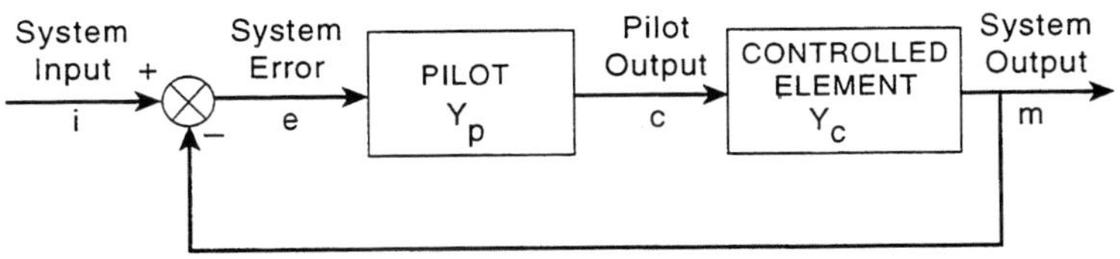

NECESSARY AND SUFFICIENT CONDITION FOR INSTABILITY

Transfer Characterics of Pilot + Controlled element

$$Y_p Y_c = -1$$

UNUSUAL CONDITIONS OF ONSET

High Gain or Task Urgency – Often with a Precursor Trigger

TYPICAL TRACKING TASKS WITH HIGH PILOT GAIN/URGENCY

- Aerial Refueling
- Formation Flying
- Precision Tracking
- Precision Approaches and Spot Landings
  (e.g., carrier approach and helicopter slope landing)
- Terrain Following
- Demanding or Unexpected Transitions

FIGURE 1-3 Conditions associated with oscillatory APCs. Source: Adapted from McRuer.[42]

which can be caused by wind gusts, turbulence, or other unexpected events (e.g., runway incursions) in the external environment. Triggers may also derive from transitional changes in the pilot or the effective aircraft. That is, transitions in the system or system elements may trigger APC events as well as change the effective aircraft or controlled element dynamics.

The essential elements that interact unfavorably to create a severe APC event (see Figure 1-4) are listed below:

- a pilot using one of several possible dynamic behavioral modes (see Chapter 5) to satisfy highly demanding tasks and goals
- less than optimum controlled-element dynamic characteristics
- triggering event(s)

HISTORICAL ANTECEDENTS

Aircraft with Conventional Flight Control Systems

The committee assessed the historical record of aircraft accidents and incidents from publicly available records and detailed discussions with a representative set of aircraft manufacturers, airlines, and accident investigation authorities in the United States and Europe. This assessment revealed a remarkably diverse set of severe PIOs and other APC events. Tables 1-1a through 1-1d show a cross section of PIOs for aircraft that are considered classical and traditional from the standpoint of FCSs. Although these include some very current aircraft, with few exceptions the FCSs comprise conventional mechanical primary controls that connect the pilot to hydraulically-actuated control surface effectors. These primary control systems are usually supplemented with relatively simple, restricted authority SASs that were added to improve the effective aircraft dynamics.

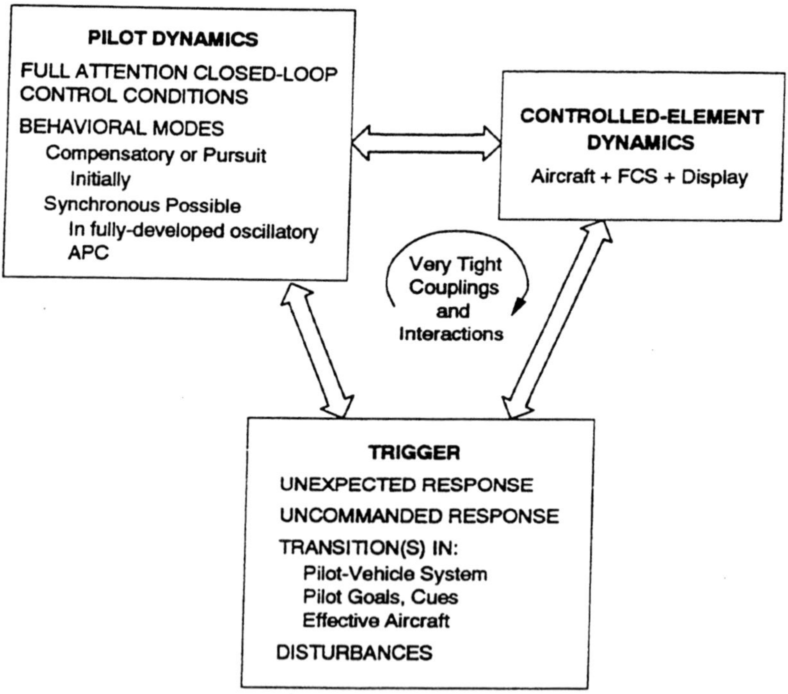

FIGURE 1-4 Interacting constituents of oscillatory APCs.

TABLE 1-1a Single Axis PIOs Associated with Extended Rigid Body Effective Aircraft Dynamics

Aircraft	Date	Description
XS-1	Oct. 24, 1947	PIO during gliding flight approach and landing
XF-89A	Early 1949	PIO during dive recovery
Mirage	1950s	Several severe pitch PIOs on early aircraft with FCSs not equipped with a pitch-damping system
KC-135A	late 1950s	Mild lateral-directional PIO associated with lateral-directional coupling effects
X-15	June 8, 1959	PIO during gliding flight approach and landing
X-15	1961	Lateral PIOs during research study of lateral-directional coupling
Parasev	1962	Lateral rocking PIO of paraglider research vehicle during ground tow
B-58	Sept. 14, 1962	Lateral-directional, control-associated PIO resulting in a crash
M2-F2	May 10, 1967	Lifting body, lateral-directional PIO
MRCA	1975	Short take off PIO
	1976	Heavy landing PIO
MD-11	April 6, 1993	PIO following inadvertent deployment of slats

[a] Category I, II, and III PIOs are defined in Chapter 2.
Source: Adapted from McRuer.[42]

TABLE 1-1b Single-Axis PIOs Associated with Extended Rigid Body Plus Mechanical Elaborations

Aircraft	Date	Description
A4D-2	Jan. 19, 1957	High-speed Category III PIO during routine flight testing involving the bobweight effect* and the primary control system
F8U-1	1957	PIOs occurred when fuselage bending caused anomalous inputs to FCS pitch axis control (referred to as a "walking beam" problem), which exaggerated the pilot's commands, especially at high speed and low altitude
T-38	Jan. 26, 1960	High-speed Category III PIO, involving the bobweight effect and the primary control system (see Figure 1-1)
F-4	May 18, 1961	Destructive PIO during an attempt to set a low-altitude speed record

Source: Adapted from McRuer.[42]

TABLE 1-1c Single-Axis, Higher-Frequency PIOs

Aircraft	Date	Description
YF-12	Several incidents in late 1960s and early 1970s	PIO involving high-frequency flexible modes of the airframe structure
CH-53E	1978–1985	PIOs involving flexible modes during precision hover with heavy sling loads, which resulted in heavy landings and dropped loads
F-111	unknown	Several PIO incidents caused by coupling of the pilot with heavy underwing stores, which resulted in sustained lateral oscillations
Voyager	1986	PIOs caused by coupling of the pilot with symmetric bending of the wing

Source: Adapted from McRuer.[42]

TABLE 1-1d Combined Three-Dimensional, Multi-Axis PIOs

Aircraft	Date	Description
X-5	Mar. 31, 1952	Three-axis PIO leading to crash
AD-1	Several incidents in early 1980s	Three-axis PIOs associated with inherent couplings of oblique wing aircraft
F-14	Jan. or Feb. 1991	PIO with high angle of attack (α) with some sideslip angle (β)

Source: McRuer.[42]

PIOs in Tables 1-1a through 1-1d are divided by two distinguishing features into four groups, each exemplified by well-known incidents (some of them catastrophic). The two primary features are: (1) the number of aircraft control axes involved in the PIOs; and (2) the frequency of oscillation of the closed-loop PIOs. The number of aircraft control axes is defined as the number of vehicle command variables the pilot was using to control the aircraft at the time of the PIO. For example, control of pitch motions using the elevator would correspond to one control axis, whereas pitch control effected by the elevator, ailerons, and rudder would correspond to three axes. The frequency range over which control is exerted can vary from about 0.2 to 3 Hz. At the higher frequencies the flexible modes of the aircraft play an important role in the PIO. In the lower frequency regime, say 0.2 to 1 Hz, the effective aircraft dynamics are basically the dynamics of the aircraft as a rigid body modified by the low-frequency effects of higher-frequency FCS components, including actuation elements; these are referred to as "extended rigid body dynamics."

Many APC events in Tables 1-1a through 1-1d are not well documented. Several occurred on research aircraft that presented state-of-the-art stability and control challenges; these PIOs have helped to define the limits of piloted control and have underscored the need for sophisticated FCSs to redress imbalances in certain configurations. For those aircraft that were already operational or that became operational, the specific problems leading to PIOs were identified, and the aircraft were modified to reduce PIO tendencies. This was accomplished largely on an ad hoc basis and usually required extensive flight testing. Solutions and fixes have been guided by flying qualities research aimed at developing requirements for military aircraft, by major developments in pilot-vehicle analysis that improved understanding, and by after-the-fact simulation.

Aircraft with Fly-by-Wire Flight Control Systems

Table 1-2 shows some PIO and non-oscillatory APC events associated with FBW aircraft. The entries in this table differ in several ways from those in Table 1-1. First, not all of the incidents are as well known as those in Table 1-1. Second, all the aircraft in Table 1-2 are modern. Third, and finally, incidents in the development phase of new commercial transports are included. The common attribute of the aircraft in Table 1-2 is that they are all equipped with modern FBW FCSs. As a matter of historical fact, almost every aircraft with a partial or total FBW FCS (including the Shuttle orbiter, F-16, F-18, YF-22, B-2, C-17, A-320, Boeing 777, and JAS-39) has, at one time or another in the development process, experienced one or more APC events. The new FBW era may be a historical watershed in that, although many FBW aircraft have been enormously successful in the production phase by virtue of the advantages conferred by FBW technology, all of them have passed through a period of APC difficulties.

It is now generally accepted that FBW technology, which in this report includes fly-by-light* technology, offers many opportunities for new solutions to aircraft stability and control problems of all kinds. The introduction of FBW systems technology has also created systems with enormous advantages in terms of performance, weight reductions, stability and control, operational flexibility, and maintenance requirements. At the same time, almost as a corollary, the flexibility inherent in FBW technology introduces more opportunities for new side effects and unanticipated problems. The counterpoint, however, is that FBW technology also offers a great many possibilities for correcting problems. This benefit has been amply demonstrated by experience in correcting the problems documented in Table 1-2. The flurry of APCs encountered in modern aircraft development programs suggests that, although FBW systems are not inherently more or less susceptible to severe APC events, the technology is new, and some side effects have not been fully explored.

TABLE 1-2 Noteworthy APC Events Involving FBW Aircraft

Aircraft	Date	Description
YF-16	1974	Unplanned first flight during a high-speed taxi test
Tornado	Jan. 26, 1976	Landing accident during flight test of prototype #5
Shuttle	Oct. 26, 1977	Flight ALT-5 (Approach and Landing Task 5): Category II PIO during landing approach glide; both attitude and path modes involved
DFBW F-8	April 18, 1978	Category III PIO during touch-and-go landing and takeoff exercise
F-18	1970s	PIO during air-to-air refueling tests of early version of flight control system
A-320	1980s	Several undocumented PIOs that reportedly occurred during development
JAS-39	1990	Category II or III PIO during approach
	1993	APC event during low altitude flight demonstration
YF-22	April 25, 1992	Category III PIO after aborted landing prior to touchdown
C-17	1988–1994	A variety of oscillatory phenomena were encountered during several phases of the development process: fixed-base simulation, motion-based simulation, "iron-bird" simulation, and flight testing
V-22	1994	Pilot involvement with the following: • 1.4 Hz lateral oscillation on the landing gear • 3.4 Hz antisymmetric mode destabilized by pilot aileron control • 4.2 Hz symmetric mode destabilized by pilot collective control
B-2	1994	APC events during approach and landing and aerial refueling
B-777	1995	Several PIOs during development flight test: • pitch oscillations at touchdown triggered by deployment of spoilers • pilot's use of a pulsing technique to control pitch excited a 3-Hz flexible bending mode • oscillations after takeoff triggered by a mistrimmed stabilizer

Source: Adapted from Dornheim,[12] McRuer,[42] NTSB.[51]

STUDY OVERVIEW

The National Aeronautics and Space Administration (NASA) asked the National Research Council (NRC) to conduct a study to determine the current status of APC problems as a potential safety issue. This study, under the auspices of the Aeronautics and Space Engineering Board, focuses attention on key steps that could be taken to minimize the kind of problems seen recently and that could counter new types of APC events.

Statement of Task and Committee Membership

To fulfill this assignment the Aeronautics and Space Engineering Board assembled the Committee on the Effects of Aircraft-Pilot Coupling on Flight Safety. Committee members have expertise in the technical, operational, and safety disciplines associated with PVSs (see Appendix A for biographical sketches). The NRC charged the committee to evaluate the current state of knowledge about APC events and to recommend processes that may help eliminate adverse APC tendencies from military and commercial aircraft. The statement of task asked the committee to do the following:

- Review and assess recent incidents and accidents in which adverse APC is known or suspected.
- Review current and projected FBW and fly-by-light applications with emphasis on potential APC issues.
- Evaluate current processes for ensuring that APC characteristics of current and future aircraft do not constitute undue safety risks and, if appropriate, recommend improvements in these processes.
- Assess the current scope, depth, and balance of national and international efforts devoted to the resolution of problems involving APC and define key areas and issues of concern.

The committee received significant help from technical liaisons from NASA, the U.S. Navy, the U.S. Army, and the Federal Aviation Administration (FAA), as well as many national and international experts who expanded and augmented the committee's expertise (see Appendix B).

Study Approach

As described above, adverse APC is a systems problem that occurs when human behavior and effective aircraft dynamics interact in peculiar ways. Human pilot dynamic behavior and aircraft/FCS dynamics are highly complex technical disciplines that are ordinarily treated by a three-pronged approach—analysis, computer simulation, and experiment. Like other problems of overall systems engineering, this one requires systems-level thinking and intimate knowledge of the system details.

The committee was also challenged with finding understandable and straightforward language (in fields replete with jargon) to communicate with a community that has diverse interests, needs, and time horizons. The anticipated audience for this report includes technical, government, and administrative decision makers and their technical and administrative support staffs; key technical managers in the aircraft manufacturing and operational industries; stability and control engineers; aircraft FCS designers; research specialists in flight control, flying qualities, and human factors; and technically knowledgeable lay readers. On the face of it, persuasive communications with such a diverse audience is extremely difficult.

The problem of technical jargon is partly handled with a glossary. Finding an appropriate level of technical discourse was more difficult. For instance, verbal explanations of complex phenomena can only go so far without resorting to mathematically expressed analyses; credible comparisons of approaches are best expressed in graphical depictions and tabulations of data, and so on. But such techniques in a report intended to persuade technical and administrative managers and even technically knowledgeable lay readers may obscure rather than illuminate the intended message. Accordingly, the committee has attempted to produce a report that can satisfy the needs of most readers, as they were perceived by the committee. The approach adopted to achieve this end was to prepare a multifaceted, multilevel report that incorporates material of varying complexity.

The committee engaged in an international information-gathering effort that included interactions with aviation industry experts from France, Germany, Russia, Sweden, and the United Kingdom (in addition to the United States). Based on these discussions, the committee determined that the findings and recommendations contained herein are generally applicable nationally and internationally.

Report Organization

The executive summary is self-contained and provides a general explanation of APC problems and a summary of the committee's findings and recommendations.

Chapters 1 through 4 focus on new systems; APC phenomena, status, and trends; and recommended processes. Chapter 1 sets the stage with an explanation of how APC is rooted in the PVS, definitions, and historical antecedents. Chapter 2 describes the wide spectrum of APC phenomena and the underlying constituents, PIO categories, and case studies of APC-related incidents and accidents. Chapter 3 summarizes trends of adverse APC from a review of accidents and incidents, points out difficulties in the identification and analysis of operational situations, and describes the associated need to better identify APC possibilities in operational situations. Chapter 4 lists lessons learned and recommends management and design policies, procedures, and processes to avoid adverse APC events.

Chapters 5 and 6 focus on tools. Chapter 5 examines experimental and analytical techniques that can be used to discover and understand APC events and to study alternative systems. Chapter 6 compares available analytical procedures for assessing APC potential and describes the committee's conclusions related to criteria. Chapter 7 lists the committee's major findings and recommendations.

The appendices provide amplifying information in support of the main body of the report. Appendix A contains biographical sketches of committee members. Appendix B lists participants in committee meetings. Appendix C provides a detailed technical description of essentially linear oscillatory APC events and some nonlinear characteristics that lead to flying qualities "cliffs."* Appendix D describes ongoing research to mitigate APC tendencies and improve the capabilities of piloted simulations for evaluating APC problems.

2

Varieties of Aircraft-Pilot Coupling Experience

INTRODUCTION

From the pilot's perspective, aircraft-pilot interactions fall somewhere between two extremes—the pilot may be fully interactive, or the pilot may be effectively detached. In the fully interactive extreme, the pilot is said to be "in the loop," and the PVS operates as a closed-loop feedback control system. In this situation, the pilot's commands are more or less continuous and depend, at least partly, upon pilot-perceived "errors" or differences between desired and actual aircraft responses. Near the opposite extreme is the "open-loop" control system, in which the pilot operates as a forcing function, generating commands to the effective aircraft that are not directly related to the pilot's perception of aircraft motion. In either case, the PVS operations involve "aircraft-pilot interactions" that constitute an all-inclusive set.

The interactions may result in motions that are desirable and "benign" or "undesirable." For this study, the interactions of interest are primarily closed-loop in character. They can result in favorable PVS responses that converge to provide the desired PVS performance, or they can result in undesired responses, either oscillatory or divergent. The focus here is on unfavorable, closed-loop PVS responses, both oscillatory and divergent. Unfavorable responses need to be understood in the context of the all-inclusive set of all PVS operations. The hierarchical structure shown in Figure 2-1 provides a taxonomy that is useful for classifying, discussing, and analyzing APC phenomena.

At the highest level, aircraft-pilot interactions are divided into benign and undesirable. Routine piloting, which is the most prevalent form of aircraft-pilot interaction and which can involve both open-loop and closed-loop operations of the PVS, is shown on the far left of Figure 2-1 as the most benign (and desirable) class. Routine piloting includes all well-accomplished piloting tasks as well as two kinds of PVS oscillations. The first, which arises from incomplete pilot adaptation to the effective aircraft dynamics, is very common and, fortunately, usually benign. These oscillations usually occur when the pilot is adapting to the aircraft dynamics and performing high-gain, precision-control tasks. For example, 15 oscillation incidents occurred during testing of the SAAB J-35 in 1960; 7 of these occurred when a pilot was flying the J-35 for the first time.

From time to time in this learning process, the pilot's gain is momentarily high enough to create a closed-loop oscillation. The usual initial "cure" is simply for the pilot to get out of the loop by releasing the inceptor and relying on the stability of the effective aircraft dynamics to handle the recovery. Because this is basically a learning experience, the ultimate cure is practice.

The other kind of closed-loop PVS oscillations that can be considered normal is a low-amplitude, damped oscillation, which is often referred to as a "bobble." Bobbles are associated with short-duration, excessive pilot gain. They are, at worst, short-term, mild PIOs that do not cause difficulties in controlling the aircraft.

The next class of favorable and benign interactions includes oscillations deliberately introduced by the pilot to generate a periodic forcing function. The outstanding example of this is "stick pumping," when the pilot applies an oscillatory input to the aircraft either to "feel out" its effective dynamics or to counter large control-system nonlinearities (as a kind of "dithering control"). The pilot's input constitutes an open-loop forcing function, and the pilot's action and the resultant aircraft oscillation frequency are not directly conditioned by the aircraft's response.

The undesirable APC events that are the subject of this study appear in the right half of Figure 2-1. Within this group, PIOs are distinguished from non-oscillatory APC events like divergences. The oscillations are akin to the benign "learning experience" variety, but they are not associated with pilot maladaptation. In fact, the pilot may be very experienced with the aircraft and with the task in general. Sometimes, however, the task specifics suddenly become unusually severe, requiring a highly aggressive pilot response to exert precise control and regulation of the aircraft. In this situation, getting out of the closed loop is not always feasible, so the demands for recovery focus on the PVS rather than just on the effective aircraft. Forced by circumstances to retain some level of control while attempting to recover, the pilot's gain may be too high but cannot be relaxed. The result can be a severe or even catastrophic PIO even with the very best, most well adapted pilot. The pilot-vehicle closed-loop system is simply not up to the demands imposed on it.

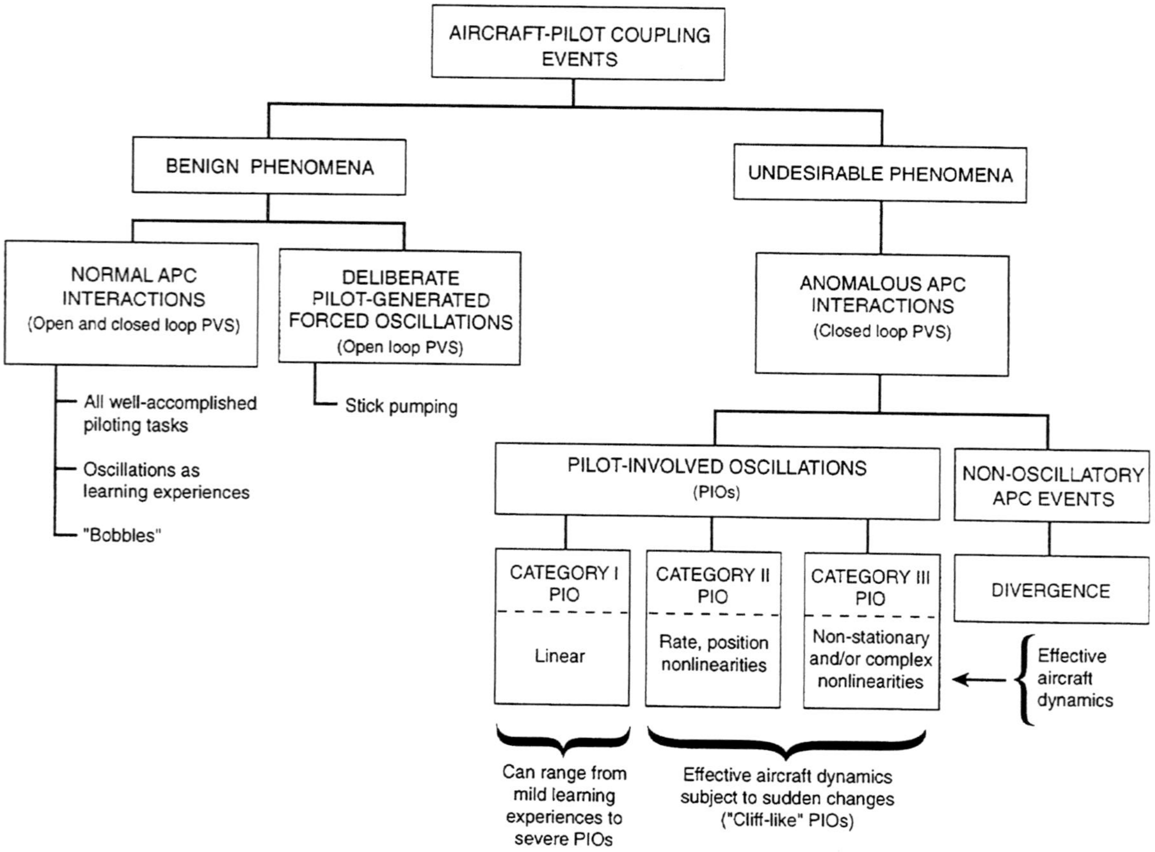

FIGURE 2-1 Taxonomy of APC phenomena.

Depending on the effective aircraft dynamics, three categories of unfavorable PIOs can be distinguished. (Each of these categories is described in more detail in the following section.) For Category I PIOs, the dynamics are essentially linear; Category II and III PIOs involve nonlinearities in the effective aircraft dynamics. In Category II PIOs, the nonlinearities result from rate or position limits (the rest of the effective aircraft dynamics are essentially linear). The nonlinear features in Category III PIOs are more complex. The nonlinear properties in both Category II and III PIOs can cause sudden changes in the effective aircraft dynamics that result in the abrupt (sometimes referred to as "cliff-like") onset of PIOs.

The class in Figure 2-1 furthest to the right comprises non-oscillatory APC events. These Category III events can stem from several causes and tend to be highly idiosyncratic. Only a very few incidents have been identified to date, but the advent of FBW technology has introduced some new dimensions by permitting control mechanizations that can be troublesome, especially in highly limiting conditions.

The next section, Categories of Aircraft-Pilot Coupling Oscillations, begins with a description of the three categories of oscillatory APCs. This description is followed by discussions of nonlinear, "cliff-like" PIOs and of non-oscillatory APC events. The next major section, Triggers, presents a fuller description of the underlying conditions and the kinds of triggers thought to be involved in initiating adverse APC events of all classes. Finally, several varieties of PIOs are illustrated by case studies. Four detailed examples are presented, along with a separate discussion of APC issues related to rotorcraft. The case studies are typical incidents and accidents encountered in the development phases of recent FBW systems. They are particularly instructive in that each exhibits a PIO in a concrete and specific context. Taken together, they provide a broad picture of a variety of potential triggers, patterns of behavior, PIO frequencies, and so on.

CATEGORIES OF OSCILLATORY AIRCRAFT-PILOT COUPLING EVENTS

Because of the diversity in control axes, frequency ranges, and other important characteristics of PIOs, several kinds of classification schemes could be used. In the discussion of historical antecedents in Chapter 1, some notable PIOs were grouped by primary control axis and PIO frequency. Analytical studies such as McRuer[42] rely on pilot behavioral models and closed-loop analysis procedures. These studies are used to elicit understanding and explain the phenomena and their associations as well as to develop and assess system modifications to reduce the potential for PIOs. The pilot models and analysis procedures are not specific to any one group in Tables 1-1a through 1-1d. This suggests that a desirable classification scheme should accommodate existing pilot behavior models, be consistent with procedures for analyzing appropriate feedback control systems, and have direct connections with the varieties of PIO as these are reflected in experimental databases for pilot and PVS dynamics, PIO experiments, etc. To fulfill these objectives, the categories described below have been adopted. The three categories organize PIOs into classes according to whether they are essentially linear, characterized by one or two common nonlinearities, or characterized by more complex and extensive nonlinear features.

Category I: Linear Pilot-Vehicle System Oscillations

In Category I PIO phenomena, the effective aircraft characteristics are essentially linear, and the pilot behavior is "quasi-linear" and "time-stationary." Quasi-linearity means that many nonlinear elements have specific input-response pairs that appear to be similar to the input-response pairs for linear systems. This similarity leads to the notion that the pilot's output response to certain inputs can be divided into two parts: (1) the response of a linear element (known as a "describing function") that is driven by the particular input; and (2) an additional quantity (called the "remnant") that is added to this response. In the PIO situation, the input is sinusoidal (or nearly so), and the pilot's output is a periodic function that constitutes the sum of (1) a sinusoid at the same frequency and (2) a remnant composed of higher harmonics. These harmonics will ordinarily be significantly attenuated as they proceed around the PVS loop, so they do not usually materially affect the input to the pilot. The causally significant part of the pilot's dynamics in the PIO is then the pilot's sinusoidal input describing function, which for a particular input amplitude acts like a linear transfer characteristic. The time-stationary aspect of the Category I PIO means simply that the effective aircraft dynamics and the pilot's dynamics do not change during the PIO.

In Category I PIOs, no significant frequency-variant nonlinearities[28] operate in the controlled element dynamics. Simple amplitude-dependent series gain changes either in the pilot gain or the controlled-element gain can be considered special cases, so such things as nonlinear stick sensitivity or shifts in pilot attention may be admissible as features consistent with a Category I event. PIOs in this category may be deliberately induced by the pilot increasing his gain, in which case the situation is easily repeatable, readily eliminated by relaxing control (lowering pilot gain), and generally not threatening. In other circumstances (for example, when there are tight flight-path constraints and major triggering events or disturbances), the pilot may not have the option of reducing gain. Those cases may produce severe Category I PIOs.

For a given pilot cue structure, analyses of Category I PIOs can reveal pilot-vehicle, closed-loop system dynamics, bandwidths,* resonance properties, etc., for nominal and PIO-based pilot gain levels, estimated pilot ratings and commentaries, and the sensitivity of closed-loop system properties to changes in the effective aircraft characteristics. The easiest feature to estimate for Category I events is the frequency range, which depends primarily on the pilot's behavior pattern (compensatory or synchronous) and the degree to which the higher-frequency dynamics of the pilot's neuromuscular system* may be involved. (Behavior patterns are well known in human-machine systems studies.[42,45]) A cross section of frequencies that have been observed appears in Table 2-1. In some PIOs, the pilot's behavior may initially be compensatory but may change to synchronous as the oscillation develops.

The two key effective-aircraft factors associated with susceptibility to an essentially linear PIO are those that unduly restrict the pilot's ability to close the PVS loop for a broad range of gains or to achieve adequate closed-loop system performance. Much of the existing data on PIOs and poor flying qualities could be used to exemplify these factors and define them more quantitatively. Some aircraft configurations and associated analytical studies are particularly well suited to detailing these factors.[5,42] Such analyses can provide a more quantitative understanding of the effects of various effective-aircraft dynamics. Appendix C compares PVS dynamic properties for two configurations with almost identical effective aircraft dynamics except for high-frequency phase lags.* Excessive phase (or time) lag is one of the two most important aircraft-associated factors in Category I PIOs because it limits both the possible range of pilot gain adjustments and the attainable crossover frequency. These limitations directly affect the closed-loop PVS bandwidth and performance. The criteria for Category I PIOs, which are examined in detail in Chapter 6, give a quantitative answer to the question of just how much lag is "excessive."

TABLE 2-1 Cross Section of Frequencies

PVS Characteristic	Typical PIO Frequencies
Compensatory (pilot closes PVS loop to minimize error)	
Extended rigid body effective aircraft and low-frequency pilot-neuromuscular system	2 to 5 rad/sec (0.3 to 0.8 Hz)
Extended rigid body effective aircraft and high-frequency pilot-neuromuscular system	10 to 20 rad/sec (1.5 to 3 Hz); (sometimes referred to as "ratchet")
Synchronous (pure gain pilot dynamics)	
Extended rigid body effective aircraft and low-frequency pilot-neuromuscular system	4 to 10 rad/sec (0.6 to 1.5 Hz)
Flexible mode effective aircraft and high-frequency pilot-neuromuscular system	6 to 20 rad/sec (1.0 to 3.0 Hz)

Source: McRuer.[42]

The other major factor in Category I PIOs is inappropriate effective aircraft gain. This can be either too high (aircraft is too sensitive to control) or too low (aircraft is too sluggish). Too-high aircraft gain is a more important factor in Category I PIOs.

Finally, it is important to reiterate that essentially linear (Category I) PIOs are not always severe. Linear PIOs are likely to occur whenever the pilot's dynamic adaptation is faulty. These PIOs can be commonplace learning experiences that disappear as the pilot becomes familiar with the aircraft's characteristics. However, linear PIOs that occur because of excessive time lag, inadequate available gain range, or both, do not disappear and can often be severe. They are likely to be encountered whenever the PVS is confronted with extreme demands, either for high-precision control or for control of large upsets or other unexpected events. Excessive time lag and inadequate available gain range are design flaws that should be eliminated as a matter of flight safety.

Category II: Quasi-Linear Pilot-Vehicle System Oscillations with Rate or Position Limiting

Category II PIOs are severe oscillations with amplitudes well into the range where rate and/or position limits become dominant. Rate limiting goes beyond the Category I scenario by adding an amplitude-dependent phase shift and by setting the amplitude of the limit cycle.* Category II events appear to be the most common jump-resonant, limit-cycle, oscillatory APC events. (An example of jump-resonance appears below in the section on Rate Limits.)

The characteristics of typical Category II PIOs are described in the discussion of rate limiting in the next section and in more detail in Appendix C. These events are classified as a separate category primarily because rate limiting is present in a large proportion of severe PIOs. Rate limiting can be analyzed readily, and it is, perhaps, the most easily identifiable cause of a flying qualities cliff. Category II is a transitional category between Category I PIOs and the most general, nonlinear Category III PIOs.

Category III: Nonlinear Pilot-Vehicle System Oscillations with Transitions

Category III PIOs depend fundamentally on nonlinear transitions in either the controlled element or the pilot's behavioral dynamics. Shifts in the controlled element can be associated with the magnitude of the pilot's commands (akin to the rate limiting onset property in Category II). Category III PIOs may also result from a change of mode, from other internal changes in the FCS, or from changes in the aerodynamic or propulsion configuration of the aircraft.

Category III PIOs can be much more complicated than Category I or II PIOs because they necessarily involve transitions in the dynamics of either the pilot or the effective aircraft. Thus, a minimum of two sets of effective PVS characteristics are involved in Category III PIOs—pre-transition characteristics and post-transition characteristics. If these differ greatly, as they did in the T-38 and YF-12 incidents, very severe PIOs can occur.

NONLINEAR, CLIFF-LIKE, PILOT-INVOLVED OSCILLATIONS

For years, the test pilot community has recited a litany of anecdotal observations such as the following:

- Severe PIOs are sudden and unexpected.
- Sometimes, just moments before the explosive onset of a severe PIO, the aircraft is docile and easily controlled.
- Flying qualities cliffs are "out there" awaiting the right circumstances to appear and create havoc.

The validity of these observations is demonstrated by the historical events described in Chapter 1 and the case studies at the end of this chapter. The "cliff" metaphor is used to convey a sense of unexpected, dramatic, and excessively large motions of the aircraft. When cliff-like changes result from an incremental increase in the amplitude of the pilot's output, the PVS is not behaving like a linear system. Instead, this indicates the presence of significant nonlinearities either in the dynamics of the effective aircraft or in the pilot's behavior. The resulting PIOs are severe and exhibit rate-limited responses or other limit-based response patterns. Many, if not all, Category II and III PIOs exhibit cliff-like behavior.

An interesting and instructive example of cliff-like APC events was encountered during flight tests of an F-14 backup flight control module with significantly restricted rate limits.

> Of particular interest to fleet operators was the feasibility of inflight refueling and shipboard landing. Given the decrease in available stabilator rate from 35 to 10 degrees per second, the test team recognized the potential for APC due to rate limiting. An incremental build-up was designed, . . . progressively sampling the flying qualities at decreasing ranges from the tanker aircraft, and culminating in basket engagement. Throughout the approach to approximately 5 feet from the basket, the team was delighted to observe solid Level I handling qualities. They then confidently

> proceeded to engagement. Immediately upon probe contact, a longitudinal APC event initiated. Though the pilot immediately selected idle power and extended the speedbrakes, the ensuing departure was so violent that his aircraft was above the top of the vertical tail of the tanker and in 90-degree angle-of-bank prior to the probe separating from the basket. The photo/safety chase [aircraft] 500 feet abeam had to aggressively maneuver to preclude being struck by the test aircraft, and the refueling store was badly wrenched from its position on the tanker's wing pylon. The test team's naive reliance on incrementalism had badly failed them.[55]

The results of a later flight test during which a similar APC event occurred gave more detailed information about the sudden shift in PVS behavior, including why the buildup did not reveal the severe handling qualities cliff.

> Obvious from this second departure was a significant stab for the center of the basket *after* the probe had passed the lip of the basket. . . . the instrumentation revealed a three-fold increase in the magnitude of the pilot's longitudinal inputs in the seconds immediately prior to basket contact. In retrospect, this was attributed to a tanking technique in which the pilot flew formation off of the tanker fuselage up to within 2–3 feet of the basket. At that point, the pilot's point of reference shifted to the basket itself as he maneuvered the aircraft to seat the probe directly in the basket coupling. . . . In shifting the reference to the basket the control [precision demanded] abruptly tightened to inches [from feet], with a consequent abrupt increase in gain over that which had been required to maintain even very tight formation.[55]

These incidents reveal several features of cliff-like phenomena—sudden changes in the "architecture" of the closed-loop PVS as "constructed" or set up by the pilot and dramatic changes in the effective aircraft dynamics in response to changes in the pilot's commands. The consequence is the sudden onset of highly dangerous, closed-loop system behavior. The flight test doctrine of "incrementalism," in which potentially dangerous conditions are approached carefully and gradually can be a "cruel deceiver in obscuring PIO perils" in situations where the sudden onset of a highly nonlinear gain or phase lag can trigger an APC event.[55] It is essential that reliable test procedures be developed for discovering and exploring the nature of sudden shifts in the PVS that may contribute to severe APCs.

Common Cliff Producers

The cliff metaphor evokes a picture of sudden, large changes in aircraft motions associated with relatively slight changes in pilot activity. Such changes can only occur if there are significant nonlinearities in the PVS dynamics.

In conventional manual control systems, the most common nonlinearities are rate and position limits in surface actuators and various design features (such as preloads, thresholds, and detents) of cockpit manipulators (inceptors) that are designed to offset unavoidable frictional and other unfavorable effects. APC problems that can arise from these characteristics are well known among the cognoscenti, and major attention is invariably paid to them in design and flight testing.

The actuator rate and position limits are central matters in design; conditions under which rate limiting is likely to be encountered, as well as pilot techniques for coping with it, are well understood. On some older aircraft, rate limiting in surface actuation occurs when mechanical stops in hydraulic control valves (e.g., servo valve bottoming) limit continued movement of cockpit manipulators so the pilot may have a direct cue that rate limiting is present. Such features are not present on more modern, mechanically signaled aircraft, where valve over-travel is provided, and the cockpit crew is not aware when actuators are operating at the rate limit. In FBW designs, the crew has no physical connection at all to the actuators, so surface actuator rate limits are not directly apparent to the pilot. However, it is possible to design FBW systems that synthesize direct-control feel to the pilot, including inceptor motions that reflect automatic system commands or even the current position of the control surfaces.

In contrast to classical aircraft, FBW FCSs offer a broad range of possibilities for nonlinearities that can be easily implemented. The greater variety of system mode possibilities requires a fairly large number of nonlinear elements just to cope with shifts in FCS mode and aircraft configuration with changes in various interfaces, etc. The easy-to-mechanize aspects of digital control also provide a fertile field for the introduction of special situation-sensitive features intended to offset events that designers perceive as unfavorable. Thus, limiters are deliberately inserted after command signal integrators; and elaborate nonlinear features are used to reduce the undesirable time lags caused by integrators (e.g., integrator windup). Limiters are also used to set relative degrees of command authority for various functions to keep the rate limiting intrinsic in actuators from destabilizing the SAS (stability augmentation system).

In other words, there may be good reasons to introduce nonlinear features into the FCS using FBW technology. Unfortunately, designers do not always have a comprehensive understanding and appreciation of the accompanying side effects, not the least of which can be an enhanced susceptibility to adverse APCs. To illustrate how these nonlinear features can affect PIO potential, two examples of nonlinear features capable of producing cliff-like behavior in FBW systems are described below.

The two most common and significant nonlinear characteristics within the effective aircraft (see Figure 1-2) that affect closed-loop operations are command-path gain shaping and rate limiting. These are introduced by the FCS rather than the aerodynamics of the aircraft. Figure 2-2 shows a simplified view of these nonlinearities in a FCS-aircraft combination. In this system, rate limiters are present in several different locations.

In the primary manual control systems of yesteryear, the major source of rate limiting was fully powered, surface actuating subsystems. These are still present although they are sometimes "protected" from becoming active by pre-actuator rate limiters. Because these nonlinear features are present by design, they are adjustable, in principle. Any unintended harm they may do, such as contributing to a severe APC event, should be viewed as a design flaw.

Rate Limiting

Extensive control-surface rate limiting has been observed in most recorded severe oscillatory APC events, but the initiation of these events has often been attributed to other causes, usually excessive time lags. It is assumed that these time lags build up to a rate-limited oscillatory amplitude. This thesis is based on analogies with linear systems. Such excessive lags have been shown to result in poor flying qualities and to be major contributors to PVS oscillations. The excessive time lag thesis can be further supported by flight test demonstrations indicating there is some merit in "alternate control schemes" designed to offset the effects of time lag caused by rate limiting.[1,10,41] Detailed analyses also support the notion that rate limiting can exacerbate the effects of time lags.[3,14,15,31,39,46]

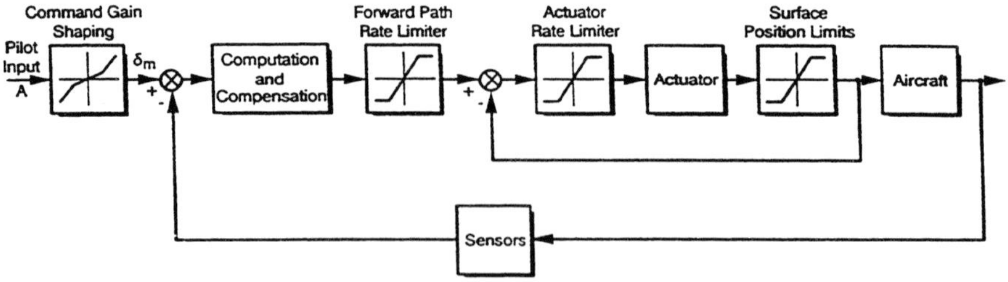

FIGURE 2-2 Most common FCS locations of command gain shaping, rate limiters, and position limiters.

Although it is clear that rate limiting phenomena are important factors in fully-developed, severe PIOs encountered in operational situations, the actual process by which rate limiting causes severe PIOs is neither well documented nor well understood. The possibility that rate limiting phenomena are primary initiating factors in the development of some severe PIOs has not received enough attention despite compelling evidence. In the F-14 example described above, for example, the sudden appearance of rate limiting features in the FCS contributed to an unexpected cliff-like situation. At its most insidious, rate limiting phenomena can cause the sudden, dramatic onset of a substantial incremental shift in the phase lag, which is instantly manifested by a change in pilot gain or command. This change is equivalent to suddenly increasing the time delay in the loop.

The general effects of rate limiting in a surface actuation system are shown in Figure 2-3. Figure 2-3a is a block diagram of a simplified surface

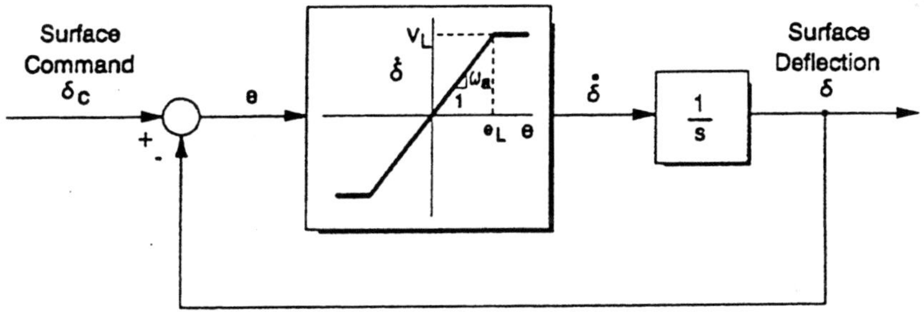

FIGURE 2-3a Surface actuator rate limiting effects for various input amplitudes in a closed-loop surface actuator system. Source: Klyde.[39]

e_L = value of e corresponding to $\dot{\delta} = V_L$

e = actuator error (i.e., the difference between the feedback signal, δ, which indicates control surface position, and the "goal position," δ_C, as indicated by the current surface command)

V_L = actuator rate limit

ω_a = bandwidth of the closed-loop actuator when operating in the linear region

1/s indicates integration

actuation system. Figure 2-3b illustrates that, for small amplitude commands, the actuator follows the command input with a small time lag (defined by the inverse of the bandwidth of the actuator as a linear system). The actuator command input, error, and output are all sinusoidal and show no effects of rate limiting. In Figure 2-3c, the amplitude of the command input is large enough to begin saturating the output velocity, but there is still little apparent effect on the output position. The time lag between input and output is essentially unchanged from the time lag of the linear system. Finally, when the command input is just a bit larger (as shown in Figure 2-3d), the actuator is rate limited (either positively or negatively) for most of the cycle. The output velocity is nearly a rectangular wave, while the output position approaches a triangular wave. Most important, the time lag between the command input and the command output is no longer even remotely related to the linear system bandwidth. Instead, it is a function solely of the rate limit and the input amplitude and frequency.

The increase in input amplitude necessary for the actuator to go from the marginal condition of Figure 2-3c to the condition of Figure 2-3d is relatively small in comparison to the input amplitude range consistent with linear operation. Thus, the onset of a significant change in phase lag can be sudden because it coincides with an increase in pilot command amplitude. From the pilot's perspective, the phase and amplitude characteristics of the actuation system change from a condition of almost no time lag (nearly pure gain) to a condition of major phase lag. In practice, this is sometimes called the "pilot overdriving the actuator," although there may be no indication to the pilot (other than an inconsistency in the aircraft's response) that the actuator is being "overdriven."

In aircraft with older versions of primary manual control systems, the onset of rate limiting may first become evident to the pilot by an increase in stick or control-column forces when the surface actuator servo valve "bottoms" (hits its internal stops). In these aircraft, the "position lag" between the pilot and the control surface seldom exceeds the valve displacement from its neutral position; as measured in degrees of control surface rotation this is typically small, on the order of 2 degrees. Thus, the pilot's output and the surface deflections are seldom far apart, and the time lag illustrated in Figure 2-3d is usually limited. Because of the mechanical connection, the sinusoidal nature of the input from the pilot shown in Figures 2-3a to 2-3d cannot be sustained except within the narrow confines of the "position lag."

The situation can be very different in more modern, mechanically signaled, primary manual control systems or in FBW FCSs; in these systems, there may be no indication whatsoever of this or other varieties of rate limiting. Therefore, the type of time lag shown in Figure 2-3d can become fully developed without being detected.

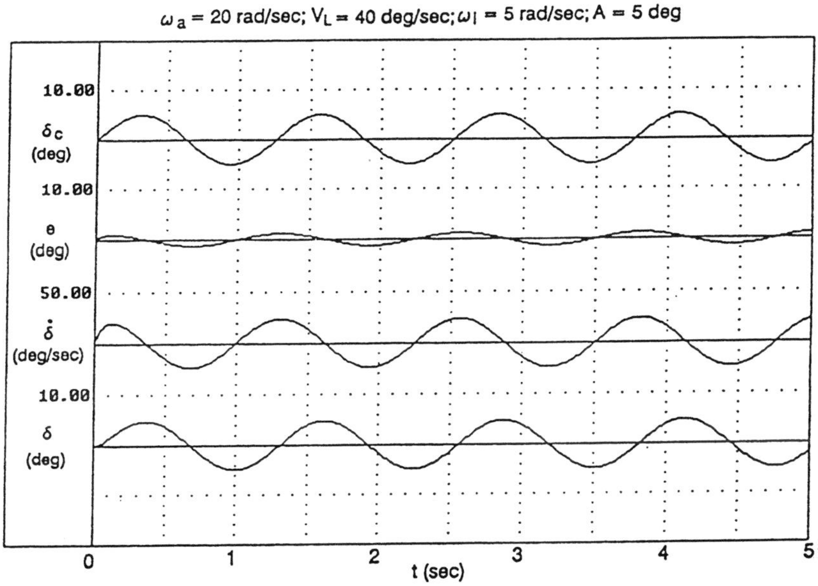

Linear System Time Responses

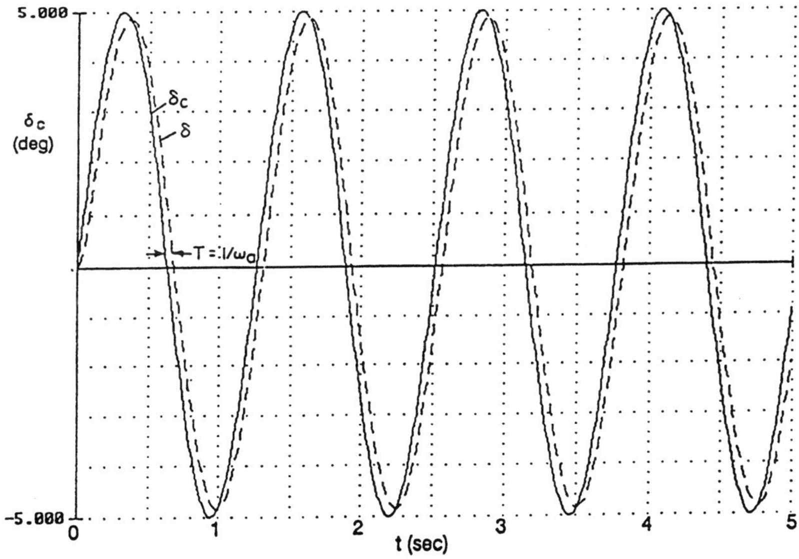

Linear System Input and Output Time Response Comparison

FIGURE 2-3b Surface actuator rate limiting effects for various input amplitudes showing linear system response times. Source: Klyde.[39]

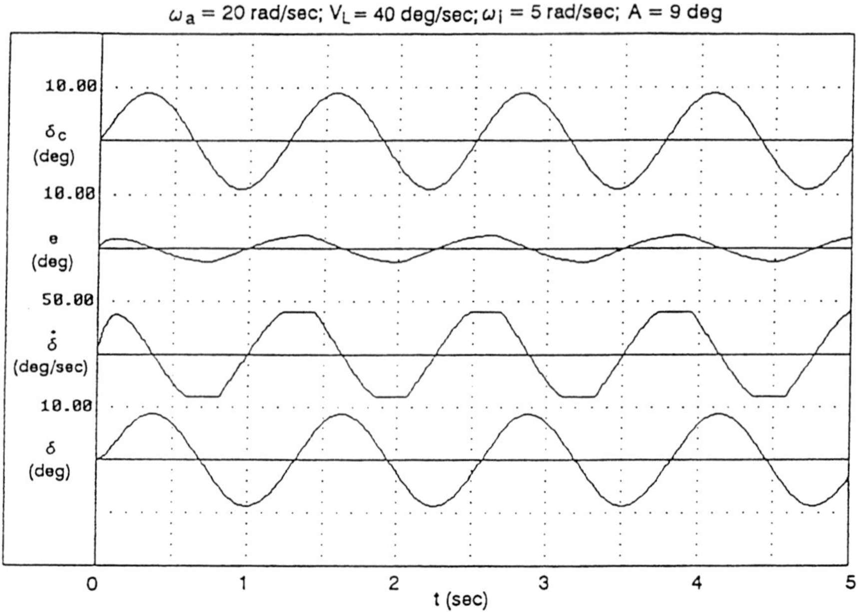

Near Saturation System Time Responses

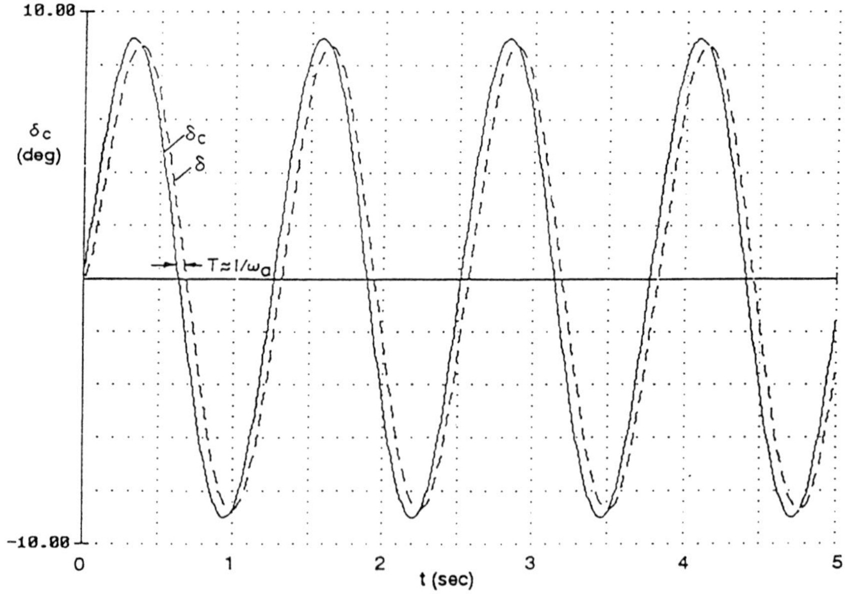

Near Saturation System Input and Output Time Response Comparison

FIGURE 2-3c Surface actuator rate limiting effects for various input amplitudes showing near saturation response times. Source: Klyde.[39]

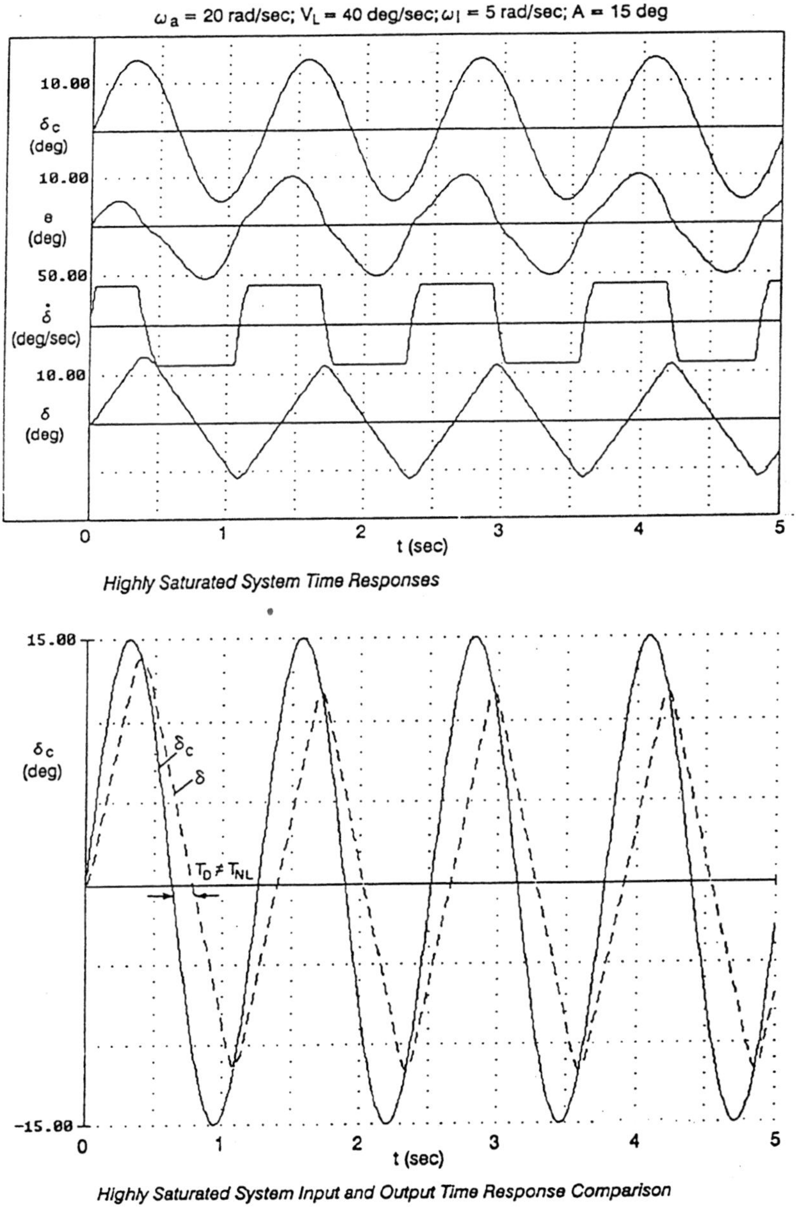

FIGURE 2-3d Surface actuator rate limiting effects for various input amplitudes showing highly saturated response times. Source: Klyde.[39]

A typical scenario begins with a pilot who is well adapted to an essentially linear, pilot-aircraft closed-loop system operating at high gain to satisfy task requirements for precision control (akin to the initial phases of the F-14 attempt to line up the refueling probe with the tanker drogue). If the pilot is confronted with task demands that call for a bit more pilot control amplitude or gain (like the pilot's attempt to finally couple with the drogue), slight increases in either pilot amplitude or gain (or both) may be sufficient to enter the nonlinear rate limiting regions, with the concomitant introduction of a sudden phase lag into the closed-loop system. In terms of the underlying physics of closed-loop systems, this is an example of a "jump resonance" phenomenon.[28]

This description suggests that rate limiting phenomena can be the main source of a flying-qualities cliff. This theory is based on the identification of rate limiting as a feature that can lead to the nonlinear oscillatory jump resonance phenomenon and is supported by studies done independently in Germany and in the United States.[3,15,39,46] The jump resonance phenomenon also emphasizes nonlinear concepts consistent with the experience of test pilots.

Jump resonance phenomena are not, of course, confined to rate limiting paradigms. An illustrative example showing rate limiting in more detail can be found in Appendix C. This example is instructive in two respects. First, the onset of rate limiting is indeed sudden and can have an immediate and substantial cliff-like effect. Second, the conditions under which onset can actually occur demand that the PVS be closed at very high gain. The PVS is assumed to be compensatory, described by the simple crossover model, with the rate limiting describing function fully developed. With these assumptions, the linear system before the onset of rate limiting has to be closed with a very high gain, corresponding to phase margins* of less than 20 degrees. When the pilot's amplitude (or gain) is increased to put the system past the onset of rate limiting, the closed-loop system immediately becomes unstable and a limit cycle is established. Similar results assuming synchronous pilot-loop closures have been obtained in another study.[17] There, a time domain simulation that demonstrated the jump resonance was used to validate frequency domain assessments that defined the onset conditions.

Because requisite circumstances are unusual, cliff-like phenomena are difficult to generate *unless* nearly exact conditions are present. In practice, this sensitivity to the conditions at onset parallels the unusual sequence that occurred with the F-14 refueling example cited above. This sensitivity also helps to explain the difficulties encountered when piloted simulations or even flight tests are used as a discovery process. The ability to analyze and pinpoint the precise conditions should make it possible to identify APC possibilities more accurately.

Command Path Gain Shaping

Almost all FBW FCSs incorporate gain shaping in the pilot's command path. Gain shaping adjusts the gain of the effective aircraft dynamics as a function of the pilot's command signal. A typical example is shown in Figure 2-4. The gain level is usually smallest for small pilot input signals. In Figure 2-4, gain shaping to provide precision control appears in the region where the absolute value of pilot input amplitude (A) is less than (a). In that region, the control gradient is equal to K_1. For larger pilot input amplitudes, the gradient increases (e.g., for $|A| > a$, the gradient increases to K_2) until maximum deflection of the control effector is achieved by maximum pilot input.

A typical APC scenario involving this nonlinear feature might start with the PVS operating with high gain to achieve precision control around neutral. In terms of Figure 2-2, the pilot's amplitude (A) for this condition does not exceed (a), although it can be very close. In the process of exerting very tight and precise control, the pilot will be closing the loop with a relatively low gain margin. (Gain margin is the ratio of the open-loop system gain for instability to the operating point gain. In a typical PVS engaged in a high-gain tracking task, experimental data indicate that the PVS gain margin will be a nominal factor of about 1.5 [in decibels this is 20 log 1.5 = 3.5 dB].[45] An increase in the open-loop system gain of 50 percent, from either the pilot or the effective aircraft, would result in neutral stability.) If a large input, a disturbance, or even-greater task demand results in a pilot output amplitude of $|A| > a$, the effective open-loop gain of the PVS increases. If the increase is sufficient to consume the gain margin, a PIO can occur. Gains with this sensitivity to pilot input have been identified as a source of severe PIOs in the past; an example is the case study of the YF-22 described below.[50] These gains can act independently or in concert with various rate limiting features.

To carry the example a bit further, a typical moderate value of K_2/K_1 in Figure 2-4 is about 3, although larger values do exist. For the high-gain PVS closure assumed here, an oscillation will occur for any pilot input of more than approximately $1^1/_3$ a, just a 33 percent increase in the input amplitude beyond the slope break-upward point.

NON-OSCILLATORY AIRCRAFT-PILOT COUPLING

In a modern FCS, the flexible attributes of FBW technology are often used to perform functions, such as alleviating the effects of wind gusts, controlling loads during aircraft maneuvers, automatically controlling the aircraft operating point, and providing stability augmentation. To accomplish these functions, the FCS often uses the same control effectors as the pilot.

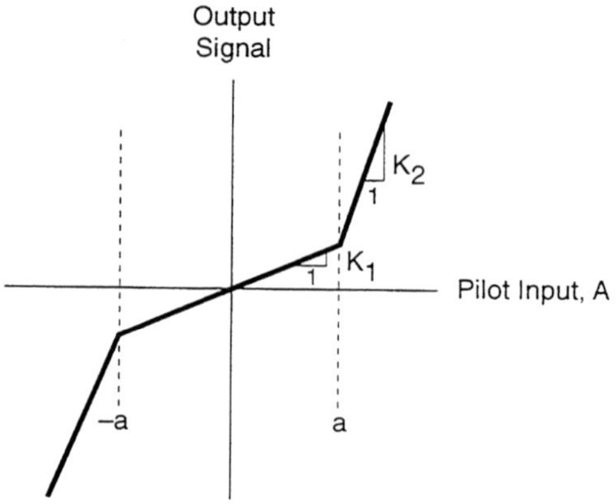

FIGURE 2-4 Example of command gain shaping for a nonlinear element. Source: Kullberg and Elgcrona.[40]

Under limiting conditions, the FCS can sometimes remove the pilot from direct access to the control effectors in order to execute these functions. Thus, the auxiliary functions can become competitive rather than cooperative. FBW controls can further interrupt the pilot's connection with the aircraft's control surfaces by introducing features such as rate limiting. If not properly accommodated and coordinated, these functions and features of the FCS can lead to great uncertainties when the aircraft is operating at and near function or surface limiting conditions.

In conventional aircraft equipped with mechanical primary controls that operate the control surfaces through a fully powered surface actuation system (and no SAS), the pilot and the control surface are mechanically connected. There is little ambiguity about where the surface is relative to the cockpit control. This state of affairs is modified when dual functions are assigned to certain control surfaces. The most common examples are "elevons," "ailevators," and "tailerons," which combine longitudinal (i.e., pitch-axis) and lateral (i.e., roll-axis) control functions into one set of control surfaces. Therefore, when one or more of the surfaces is operating at or near its limits of position, rate, or acceleration, either longitudinal or lateral control functions must be given priority. Functional allocation and priority schemes, sometimes startling in mechanical complexity, are used to this day. Of course, the reason they almost always work effectively is that they were designed with exceptional foresight to provide adequate control power for contingencies. In all cases, however, present successes are also based on a past of overlooked possibilities, surprises, fortuitous "discoveries," and ad hoc fixes and developments. Sometimes even this relatively elementary sharing of controls leads to major problems, including some of the so-called "three-dimensional PIOs" of Table 1-1.

The following APC events illustrate the kinds of problems that can occur. The first was encountered by a Tornado during a terrain-avoidance run.

> During terrain-following flight a sequence of two autopilot actions near the ground were misinterpreted by the pilot, resulting in immediate counteractions by the pilot after deactivating the autopilot. At this point the APC was fully developed. The taileron became rate saturated. Compensating for a slow roll motion, the pilot command for differential tail was not fed through to the taileron due to internal CSAS [Command Stability Augmentation System] priorities giving the pitch axis priority over the roll axis. The pilot was finally trapped into a pitch/roll APC. Manual search along the CSAS switch/control panel took the pilot out of the loop.[29]

Thus, because the pitch axis had priority, the roll was not correctable, even though the pilot may have commanded proper inputs to compensate.

An excellent, well documented example of an ultimately non-oscillatory APC is the second JAS 39 accident listed in Table 1-2.

> A time history of the second accident, which occurred during the public demonstration at the Stockholm Water Festival, is shown [in Figure 2-5]. The second accident featured a roll PIO consequent upon the pilot aggressively rolling to wings level to accelerate in front of the crowd watching the aircraft. The roll input was sufficient to drive the actuation to the deflection limit and shortly after the rate limit was reached. This caused the aircraft to roll more than expected, so the stick was reversed, driving well into the rate limiting [region] since the stick was demanding the limit of both deflection and rate. [Figure 2-6 shows] . . . the stick deflection in roll and pitch as a crossplot. With the rate limiting in effect, the inner stabilization loops were ineffective. Analysis has shown that the effective time delay between pitch stick and pitch acceleration response increased from less than 100 milliseconds to around 800 milliseconds. The subsequent response and pitch up to high angle of attack caused the pilot to eject after 5.9 seconds, fortunately without causing any harm to the crowds on the ground or the pilot.[40]

As this accident illustrates, APC problems may be complicated when additional functions share the pilot's direct authority over the control effectors.

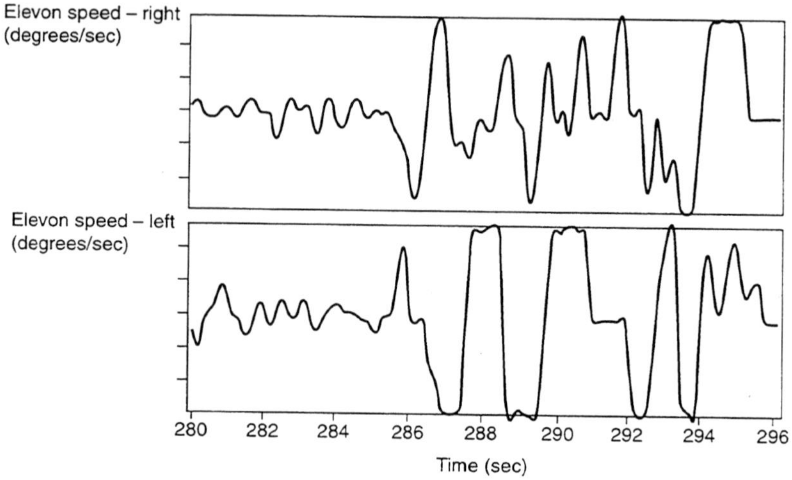

FIGURE 2-5 JAS 39 accident time history. Source: Kullberg and Elgcrona.[40]

TRIGGERS

In most cases, severe PIOs are initiated by one or more stimuli acting as triggering events. These triggers typically excite an oscillation by altering a component of the closed-loop pilot-vehicle dynamics, resulting in an unstable or very lightly damped system.

A trigger may influence the pilot, the vehicle, or both. There may be a causal chain of trigger events in which one event initiates a series of secondary triggering events (e.g., a threat of collision that results in high-gain manual control). Triggers can originate in the external environment, the vehicle, or the pilot, but all triggers have the potential to result in adverse APC that leads to aircraft upsets. Three classes of triggers are discussed below: environmental triggers, vehicle triggers, and pilot triggers.

Environmental Triggers

Environmental triggers can initiate APC events in several ways. The most direct way is an environmental circumstance that requires destabilizing control actions. One example would be a threat of imminent collision that requires large-amplitude control actions, which may result in nonlinear control response. Another example of an environmental trigger is atmospheric turbulence. Turbulence at high altitude has been linked with several severe APC events in transport aircraft.

Environmental factors can also alter the pilot's dynamics. For example, an external threat may increase the pilot's stress level, with a resulting increase in pilot gain. The external situation may also demand precision control that requires high-gain piloting, such as pitch control during landing.

Finally, environmental factors can sometimes alter the basic vehicle dynamics. For example, severe icing can alter both pitch and roll dynamics.

Vehicle Triggers

Vehicle-based triggering events most commonly involve changes in the effective aircraft dynamics that cause a mismatch between the pilot's control strategy and the aircraft dynamics. Three categories of vehicle-based triggers are discussed below.

Flight Control System-Aircraft Configuration Mismatches

A fairly common trigger, especially for a developmental PVS, is a miscalibrated FCS gain or other parameter change intended to adjust the FCS

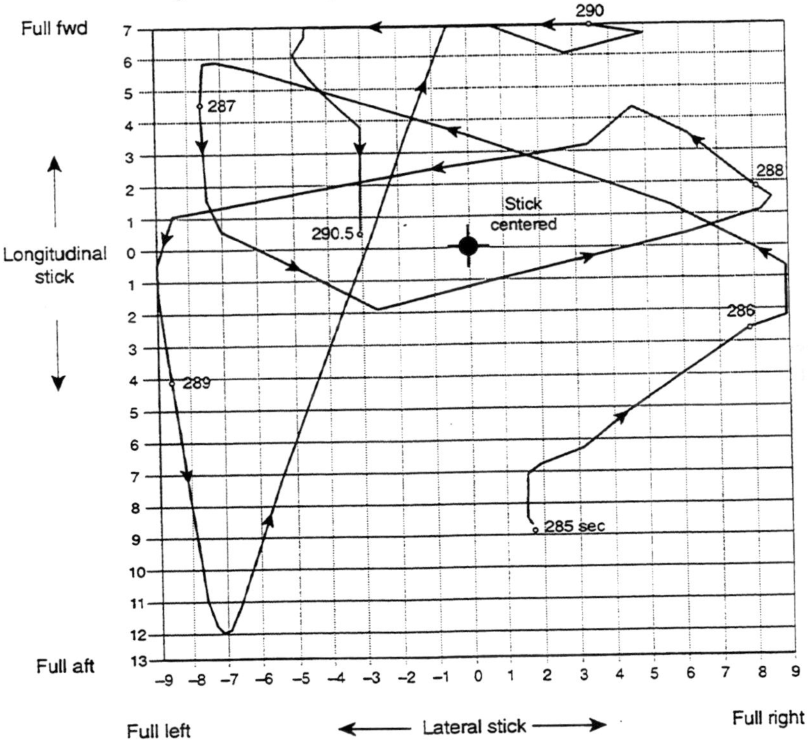

FIGURE 2-6 JAS 39 accident cross plot of stick deflection in roll and pitch during a roll PIO and unintended pitch up maneuver. Source: Kullberg and Elgcrona.[40]

properties as a function of the aircraft configuration. An example is the unanticipated level of the auto-speedbrake deployment in the Boeing 777 event (described in the Case Studies section of this chapter).

System failures

System failures can alter the effective aircraft dynamics either by changing the aircraft's response to control inputs or by changing the feedback to the pilot. Control system failures, such as failures in the hydraulic system, actuator failures, or uncontrolled changes in aircraft trim, may significantly compromise the controllability of the aircraft. Intermittent control system failures can result in highly nonlinear or discontinuous control responses that act as potential triggering events.

Sensor and display failures that alter the feedback dynamics to the pilot or the control system are also potential triggers. Even a simple mechanical failure, such as a loose pilot's seat, can alter the acceleration feedback the pilot receives and has been observed to trigger an APC event.

FCS Mode Shifts

Modern FCS technology significantly increases the ability of designers to tailor the effective aircraft dynamics for different tasks. However, it also has the potential to trigger APC events by allowing the flight control laws to change (i.e., switch modes) on the basis of numerous criteria, some of which may not be specified or understood by the pilot. If the pilot is unaware of the mode transition, a mismatch between the pilot's mental model and the effective aircraft dynamics can occur. The command path gain changes described earlier and exemplified by the YF-22 case study described later in this chapter are examples of this.

In FBW aircraft, the overall, effective response to pilot control input will depend on the inner-loop control laws and feedback gains programmed into the flight control computer. For a variety of reasons, these control laws may change during specific phases of a flight or flight conditions. For example, the "response type" in some FCSs have longitudinal stick inputs that normally command changes in the flight path angle. However, during landing operations the response type is sometimes changed so that longitudinal stick inputs command elevator position, thereby making the touchdown handling qualities more conventional. Another example (noted earlier) is the control law for the Boeing 777, which changes between "air" mode and "ground" mode. Inner-loop control law and response type transitions are usually "task tailored" to improve handling qualities. Sometimes, however, it is difficult to anticipate unusual situations where the control strategy is inconsistent with the pilot's intentions.

The lack of some inceptor-motion or other proprioceptive feedback in some FBW aircraft deprives the pilot of some "display" cues, and this lack of cues can, perhaps, trigger a Category II or III APC event. Rate limiting or other nonlinear control elements inserted after the pilot's command can introduce time lags that effectively disconnect the pilot from the aircraft, thereby leading the pilot to generate unreasonable inputs. The second JAS 39 accident discussed above is at least partly attributable to this problem.

Other new APC triggering mechanisms that have resulted from the extensive and common use of automation in modern aircraft stem from mixed-mode control. For some aircraft, it is common to fly in mixed manual and automatic control modes (e.g., pitch is controlled manually while speed is controlled by autothrottles). One mixed automation mode that has caused an APC event is the use of elevator trim for stability augmentation at high altitude. Elevator trim motions commanded by the SAS can interact with the pilot's manual inputs for controlling pitch, particularly in turbulent conditions.

Based on the available incident data, the potential for automation-related PIOs increases in situations where there is a sudden manual takeover from automated control, such as an autopilot disconnect in an out-of-trim condition. When pilots are in a supervisory status (i.e., out of the control loop), problems may arise if they are required to intervene suddenly. Slow response by the aircraft can result in inadequate control or over-control. Inappropriate mental models or incorrect situation assessment can lead to control actions that result in undesirable aircraft motion.

The manual takeover problem is exacerbated when the automation causes or masks significant changes in the underlying effective aircraft dynamics. In this case, the pilot is suddenly given a perhaps marginally stable aircraft to control. For example, degradation in lateral control during severe icing conditions is thought to have been the cause of the ATR 72 accident in Roselawn, Illinois, on October 31, 1994. The degradation was masked by the autopilot; when it was disconnected, the pilots were never able to regain stable flight. The manual takeover problem is an example of the "post-transition retention of pre-transition behavior." In this case, the transition is from automatic to manual control and the controlled element dynamics under manual control are not well modeled by the pilot.

In some cases, manual takeover problems have been combined with problems of mixed manual and automatic control modes. Examples include the China Airlines A 300-600 accident at Nagoya Airport near Tokyo on April 26, 1994, and the Tarom A 310-300 incident at Orly Airport in Paris on September 24, 1994. In the Nagoya event, the autopilot attempted to perform a go-around using the stabilizer trim while the crew attempted to fly the glide slope with the elevator. The resulting nose-up trim was so extreme that the aircraft pitched up uncontrollably when the pilot increased thrust. The accident sequence started with the pilot manually flying the aircraft, although the flight director guidance system and autothrottles were engaged to maintain speed. During the approach, the pilot inadvertently activated the autopilot takeoff/go-around switch. Several seconds later, after the pilot noted that the switch had been activated, the autothrottles were disengaged, but the autopilots were then engaged, perhaps with the expectation that the autopilots would return the aircraft to the proper glide slope for approach. Instead, the autopilots used elevator trim to establish a large nose-up pitch consistent with a go-around. At the same time, the pilot attempted manually to get the nose down and return to the approach glide slope using control column commands to the elevators. By the time the pilot disconnected the autopilot and attempted a go-around, the aircraft was so out of trim that the aircraft reached a pitch angle of 52.6 degrees, slowed to 78 knots, and stalled at an altitude of 1,800 feet. The pilot was unable to regain control.[61]

Pilot Triggers

In many APC events, the precursor or trigger is pilot-related. Often an environmental or vehicle trigger precedes the pilot trigger, and the APC event results from an overreaction or lack of appropriate reaction on the part of the pilot.

Pilot gain often increases and can become excessive as a result of task-related or situation-related stress. The pilot's concentration on particular cues to the exclusion of others is often desirable. However, excessive exclusive concentration, called "tunneling," can lead to a momentary excessive gain and, subsequently, a pilot-triggered upset. Unexpected changes lead to the most severe situations. Pilot stress can be induced by an external threat that results in an adrenaline surge. Stress can also be task-induced when the pilot attempts a high-gain, high-stress task, such as aerial refueling or aircraft-carrier landing.

Pilot-triggered APC events can also be caused by inappropriate or incorrect control strategies. Pilot-triggered PIOs are common during initial pilot training when novice pilots attempt to control the aircraft using inappropriate control variables. For example, novice helicopter pilots often attempt (unsuccessfully) to hover by controlling position directly, rather than by controlling position indirectly through attitude. One of the basic objectives of flight training is for the pilot to identify the appropriate control variables to accomplish specific manual control tasks. During training, the pilot develops a mental model of the controlled element dynamics, which is used as a basis for control strategies.

Experienced pilots may use inappropriate control strategies if they do not fully understand or appreciate the situation or they are otherwise stressed. To carry the tunneling idea further, a pilot under stress may focus on an inappropriate subset of the relevant control variables or may simply close the loop on the wrong variable.

As the complexity of modern FBW FCSs increases, the underlying effective aircraft dynamics can be task-tailored. The response type and dynamic characteristics are changed depending on a variety of criteria, such as phase of flight, airspeed, altitude, and flap settings. As the large number of potential flight-control response modes increases, so does the potential for a mismatch between the pilot's expectations of the effective aircraft dynamics and what the pilot actually experiences. If the automation is too complex, it may not be possible for the pilot to have an adequate mental model of the system. In the absence of a complete model, pilots develop ad hoc models of the effective aircraft dynamics based on nominal flight operations. In unusual or emergency situations, the pilot's ad hoc mental model of the aircraft FCS may lead to inappropriate control strategies and an increased potential for APC.

CASE STUDIES OF RECENT AIRCRAFT-PILOT COUPLING EVENTS IN FLY-BY-WIRE SYSTEMS

The following four sections describe APC events that illustrate the impact of adverse APC on developmental and operational aircraft. All four aircraft involved in these incidents used FBW FCSs. A fifth section discusses special considerations for APC events involving rotorcraft.

Case 1. Lockheed Martin/Boeing YF-22

The YF-22 is a test aircraft that was developed by Lockheed Martin and Boeing to demonstrate critical technology for the next-generation U.S. Air Force air superiority fighter. Flight testing was conducted in 1990. After the F-22 was selected for engineering and manufacturing development, additional flight evaluations were conducted on the YF-22 demonstrator aircraft in 1991 and 1992. The F-22 is scheduled for first flight in 1997.

Description of Event

On April 25, 1992, a YF-22 test aircraft was returning to Edwards Air Force Base after completing a test flight. As part of a planned photo session, the pilot performed an uneventful low approach and initiated a go-around, selecting military power and raising the landing gear. He then flew a closed pattern for a second low approach and initiated a second go-around, this time selecting afterburners. Upon raising the landing gear for the second go-around, the aircraft began a series of pitch oscillations at an altitude of approximately 40 feet. After four or five oscillations, the aircraft impacted the runway. The pilot safely evacuated the aircraft after it came to a stop, but the aircraft was destroyed.

The flight data presented in Figure 2-7 indicate the following details of this PIO:

- The PIO frequency was approximately 0.67 Hz (4.2 rad/sec).
- Neither the horizontal tail nor the thrust-vectoring nozzles were position limited during the PIO, but they did exhibit extensive rate limiting.
- The horizontal tail reached a maximum deflection of approximately ±20 degrees, and it was rate limited at 60 degrees/sec.
- The thrust-vectoring nozzles reached a maximum deflection of approximately ±14 degrees, and they were rate limited at 40 degrees/sec.
- The aircraft experienced maximum pitch rates of approximately +17 degrees/sec and −26 degrees/sec, and maximum pitch acceleration of ±90 degrees/sec^2.
- The response of the thrust-vectoring nozzle lagged behind the response of the horizontal tail by about 0.1 sec.
- There was no significant phase difference between the position of the thrust-vectoring nozzle and the pitch acceleration.
- The time difference between maxima (or minima) in pitch and pitch rate was approximately 0.45 sec. This corresponds to about 101 degrees, which is close to the expected 90 degrees (because the pitch rate is the derivative of pitch attitude for wings-level flight).
- The pitch rate lagged behind the horizontal tail position by approximately 92 degrees in the PIO. (This lag is expected to be about 90 degrees because the pitch acceleration is almost in phase with the horizontal tail, and pitch rate is simply the integration of pitch acceleration.)

Analysis

As with many APC events, the pilot initially thought that an aircraft failure had occurred. However, detailed analysis revealed that there had been no aircraft malfunction. Instead, it was determined that this event was triggered by an automatic change in pitch command gradients during the transition from gear-down to gear-up. This conclusion is substantiated by the flight recording for this accident. As illustrated in Figure 2-7, curve 2 shows a large increase in pitch rate response after the gear was raised at t = 2 sec.

Note that the large oscillations in pitch rate (curve 2), pitch attitude (curve 3), and normal acceleration (curve 4) start shortly after the gear is raised. The triangular wave appearance of curve 5, which depicts the position of the horizontal tail, indicates that the horizontal tail was essentially rate-limited throughout the event. In addition, the thrust-vectoring nozzle (curve 6) was also rate limited.

The YF-22 command gradients were largely developed in response to specific program objectives. For example, the thrust-vectoring control laws were optimized for high angle-of-attack flying qualities at high altitudes. In particular, the nose-down gradient was set to provide rapid nose-down recoveries from post-stall angles of attack.

The YF-22 control laws were not designed or analyzed for low-altitude, low-speed conditions with thrust vectoring engaged. Therefore, flight test procedures required that vectoring be turned off at low altitude. However, the flight test team did not comply with this restriction. Thus, on the second go-around, when the pilot raised the gear with thrust vectoring engaged, he unexpectedly encountered command gradients that were significantly larger than those intended for low-altitude, low-speed flight (see Figure 2-8). As a result of these large gradients, flight test data indicate that relatively small pitch stick movements by the pilot immediately prior to the PIO resulted in near-rate limiting of the horizontal tails. (A gain shift in the effective aircraft dynamics as a major source of the PIO is consistent with the analysis of command gain-shaping in Appendix C and in the section above on nonlinear, cliff-like PIOs). Thus, this PIO appears to involve the presence of (1) nonlinearities in the command path gain-shaping; and (2) nonlinear effects caused by rate limiting of the horizontal tail and the thrust-vectoring nozzle. The basic trigger was the unexpected change in pitch command gradients.

After the accident, the investigation team and the aircraft designers conducted separate evaluations of the YF-22 linear handling qualities metrics; the investigations conducted fast Fourier transform analyses to develop the pitch-attitude-to-pitch-stick frequency response* so that linear analysis such as the Aircraft-Bandwidth/Phase Delay, and Smith–Geddes Attitude-Dominant Type III criteria (see Chapter 6) could be used to determine the cause of the event. The linear analyses indicated that the YF-22 might have been susceptible to APC events with thrust vectoring engaged at low altitude. However, this conclusion has been questioned because of uncertainties about technical aspects of the analysis. For example, the coherence of the accident flight data used to generate the frequency response of the aircraft was not satisfactory because of the nonlinearity of the input signals and the rate limiting of the control surfaces.[32]

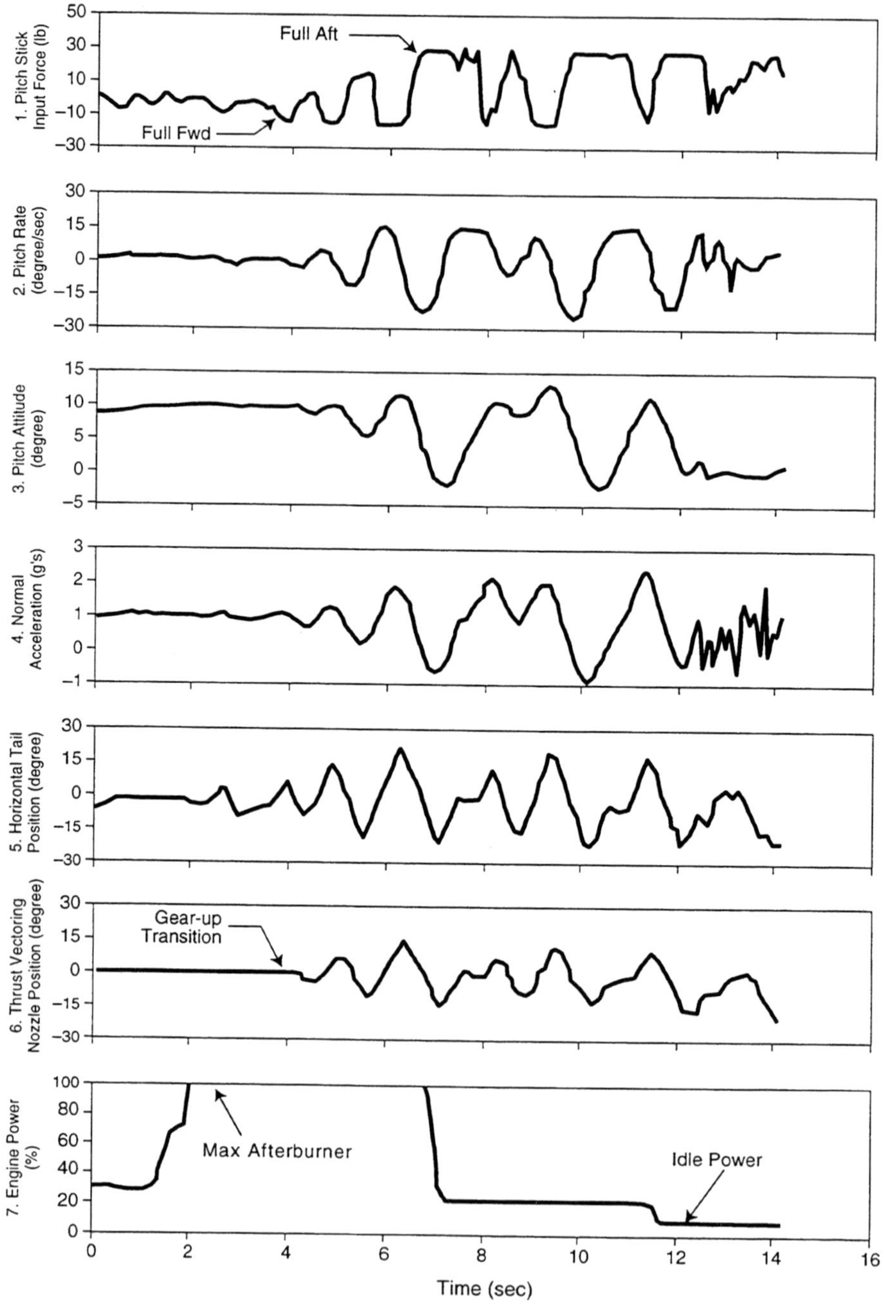

FIGURE 2-7 YF-22 accident time history. Source: Harris.[32]

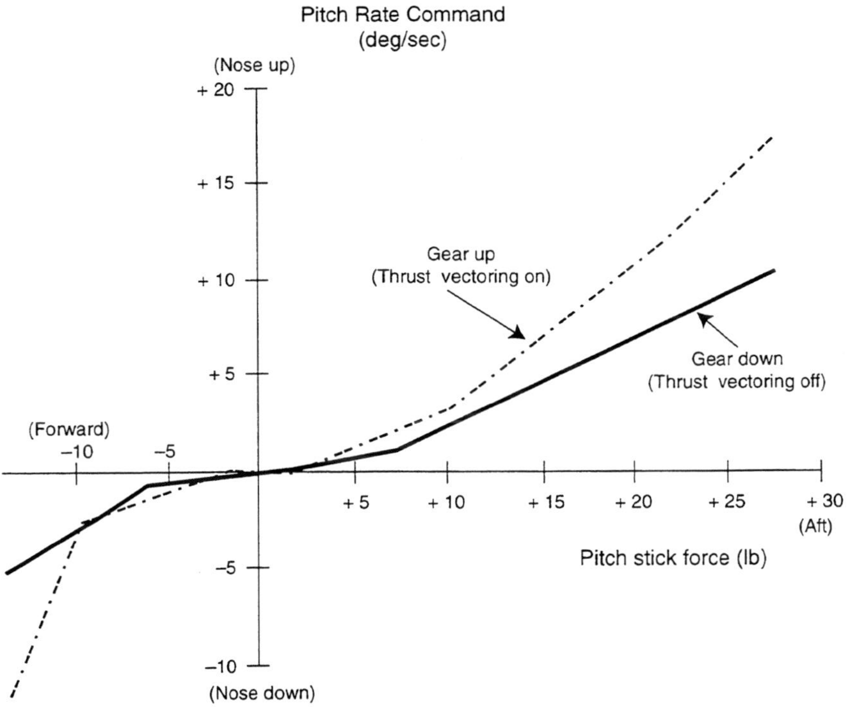

FIGURE 2-8 YF-22 pitch rate command stick gradients. Source: Harris.[32]

Post-Event Simulations

The accident review team attempted to recreate the YF-22 event using off-line and fixed-base pilot-in-the-loop simulators, but piloted simulations were unable to recreate the APC event.[32]

Case 2. Boeing 777

The Boeing 777 is a twin-engine, wide-body commercial transport with a typical seating capacity of 375. The 777 entered service in 1995, and as of January 1997, 45 aircraft had been delivered.

Description of Event

On July 24, 1994, during the thirty-fifth landing of the 777 developmental flight test program, a 777 airplane experienced an unusual PIO at the air-ground interface. Following touchdown, deployment of the auto-speedbrake generated a vertical plunge and pitch down (see Figure 2-9, curve 3) that was checked by a rapid airplane-nose-up column input (Figure 2-9, curve 1). Airplane pitch response to this column input was excessive (Figure 2-9, curve 3) and caused the pilot to make a rapid airplane-nose-down column input. This cycle continued twice more before being terminated by a combination of intervention by the other pilot and nose gear contact with the runway. A similar incident (not shown) occurred later the same day following manual speedbrake deployment.

The flight data presented in Figure 2-9 indicate that the PIO frequency is 0.40 Hz (2.5 rad/sec) and the maximum travel of the elevators is approximately +25 degrees/–30 degrees. During the event, the elevators were rate limited at +40 degrees/sec to –45 degrees/sec, the aircraft experienced maximum pitch rates of approximately +3.9 degrees/sec and –6.1 degrees/sec; the time difference between elevator position and pitch maxima or minima was approximately 1.4 sec, which corresponds to a phase shift of 200 degrees; and the time difference between elevator position and pitch rate maxima or minima was approximately 0.6 sec, corresponding to a phase difference of 86 degrees.

Post-Event Flight Test and Simulation

As a result of the initial investigation into these incidents, the sequencing for on-ground speedbrake deployment was tuned to mitigate the plunge/pitch upset that had triggered them. Also, the management of the C*U integrator* in the elevator command path (see Figure 2-10) was modified to eliminate the delay observed when large-displacement column inputs reversed direction. A flight test investigation was then conducted to identify the source of the PIO susceptibility. The maneuver that was found most effective in reproducing the PIO behavior was on-runway attitude tracking. Following touchdown, the pilot was instructed to aggressively capture and hold a target pitch attitude on the primary flight display.

Figure 2-11 illustrates the first attempt to perform this maneuver in normal mode. A small Category I (linear) PIO developed when the pilot was closing the loop on pitch attitude, making the precision capture of a specified attitude extremely difficult. The maneuver was repeated in secondary mode and found to be much easier, with no unintended oscillations (Figure 2-12). Secondary mode pitch control consists of conventional column/elevator gearing with pitch rate feedback; the C*U terms in Figure 2-10 are not present. (During landing derotation in normal mode, the control law stays "in-air" until attitude passes below a specified threshold.) The results of these tests suggest that the C*U integrator terms were the prime contributors to the derotation instability; the speedbrake pitch/plunge upset was the trigger that caused the underlying Category I APC characteristic seen in this test to become a full-

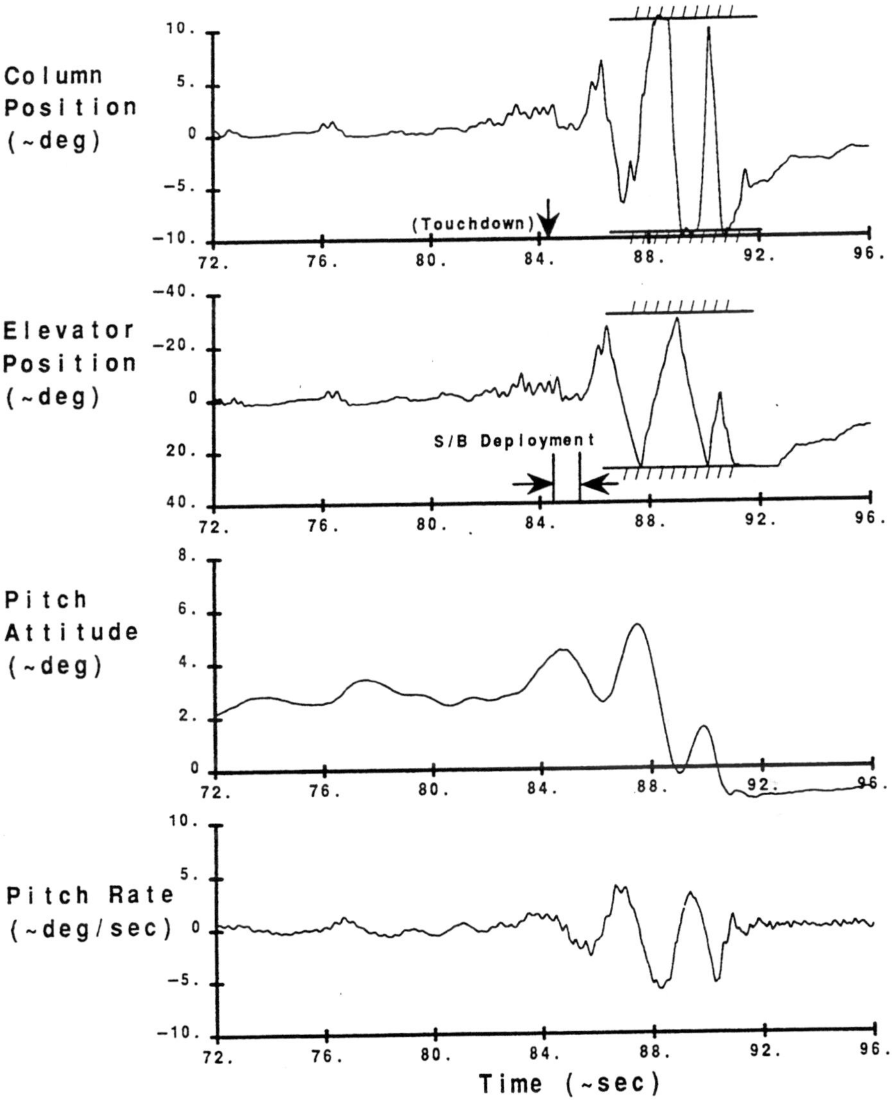

FIGURE 2-9 Time history for 777 landing derotation, baseline control law. Source: McWha.[47]

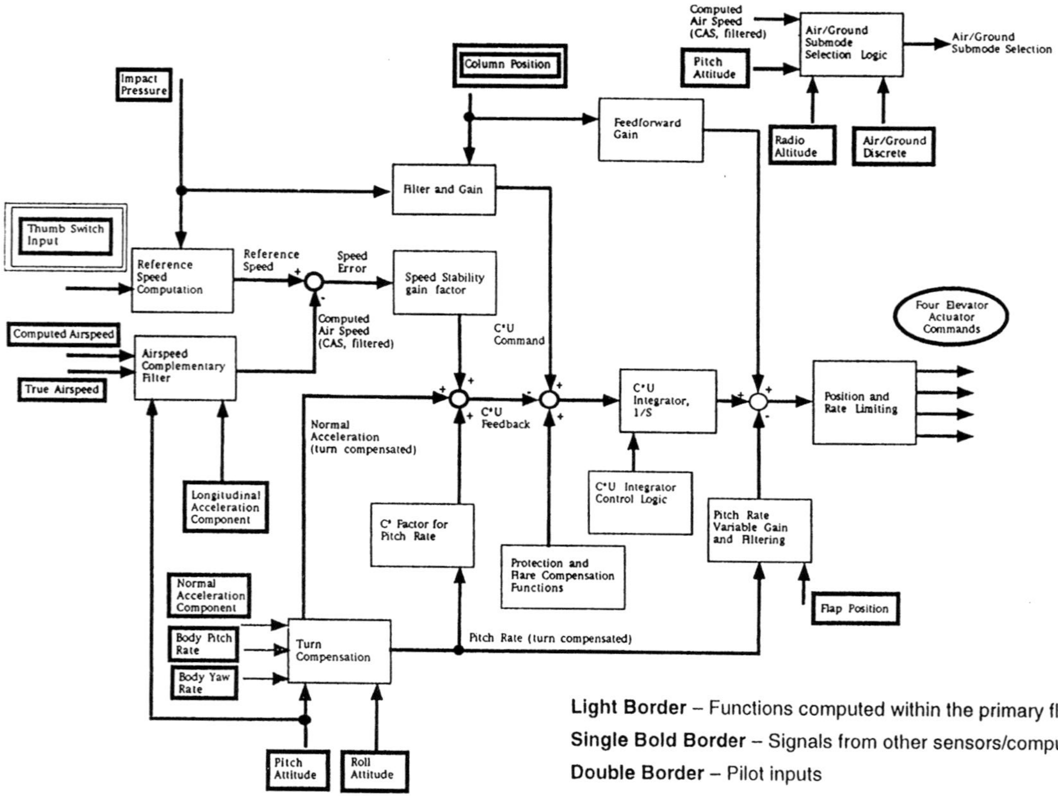

Light Border – Functions computed within the primary flight computer

Single Bold Border – Signals from other sensors/computers in the airplane

Double Border – Pilot inputs

FIGURE 2-10 Normal mode elevator control law. Source: McWha.[47]

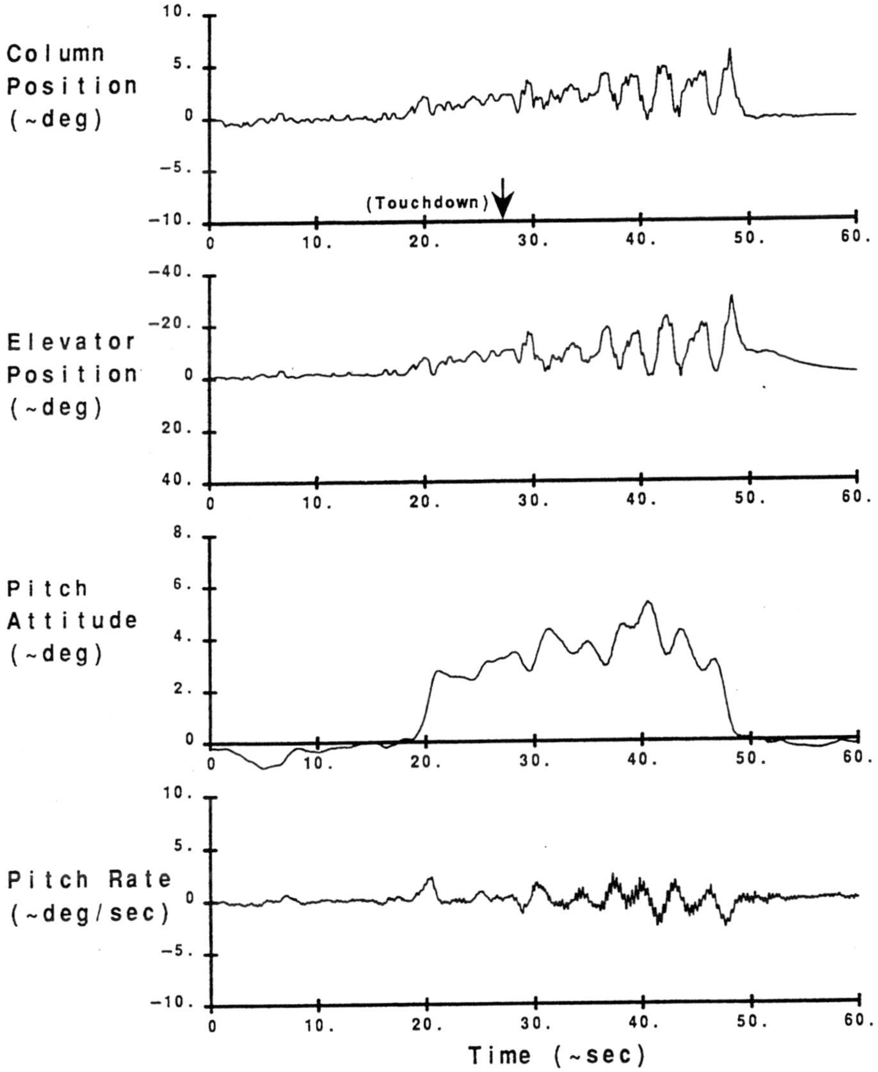

FIGURE 2-11 Time history for 777 attitude tracking on runway, baseline control law. Source: McWha.[47]

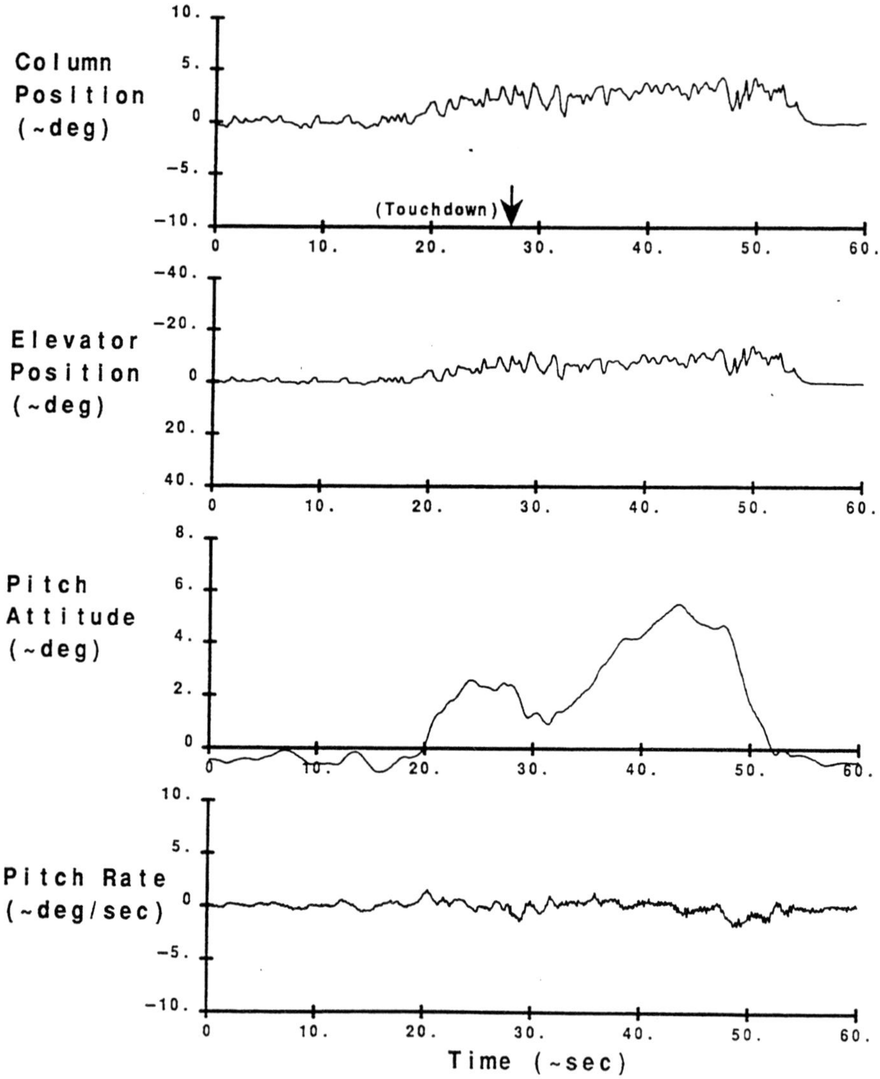

FIGURE 2-12 Time history for 777 attitude tracking on runway, secondary mode. Source: McWha.[47]

blown Category II APC event. Normal acceleration cues sensed by the pilot may have aggravated the problem.

After the flight tests and subsequent analysis, piloted simulator sessions were conducted in the 777 fixed-base simulator, which reproduced the characteristic shown in Figure 2-11. It should be noted that in the fixed-base simulator, the characteristic was manifested to the pilot in higher workload* and poorer task performance, not "PIO." Further work led to a scheme to reduce the C*U integrator gain from a nominal value of 8.0 to 3.0 at touchdown. Validation of this scheme was conducted on the airplane, which repeated much of the earlier PIO investigation test conditions. In this test, normal mode on-runway attitude tracking was found to be significantly improved. Figure 2-13 illustrates the results of one portion of this test. In this example, the pilot progressively captured 7.5, then 6.0, then 5.0 degrees, with control considered positive throughout.

Implementation of a column feed forward command notch filter motivated a final round of tracking task tests, using the same on-runway maneuver described above. Figure 2-14 contains a time history showing two pilot captures of 6-degree pitch attitude. Again, control was considered positive.

Analysis

Spectral analysis was used to assess potential control law changes. Column-to-pitch rate and column-to-pitch attitude frequency response data for the four time histories shown in figures 2-11 through 2-14 are contained in Figure 2-15. The spectral analysis for these conditions was limited to the on-runway portion of the time histories, with the nose gear off the ground and the speedbrakes fully deployed. These data show significantly less bandwidth for the original normal mode configuration than with the secondary mode or the later normal mode configurations. Note that the 180-degree frequency for the original PIO-prone normal mode configuration is essentially the same as the observed PIO frequency in Figure 2-11.

Another way of looking at the pitch control system characteristics, which was found to be useful for on-ground operation, was to examine the net column-to-elevator gearing and phase behavior. Figure 2-16 contains column position to elevator position frequency response data from the same time histories. The original normal mode configuration is seen to have excessive gain at low frequencies, with significantly greater phase lag than the secondary mode or the later normal mode configurations. This additional elevator activity was caused by the C*U integrator acting at the original high-gain values.

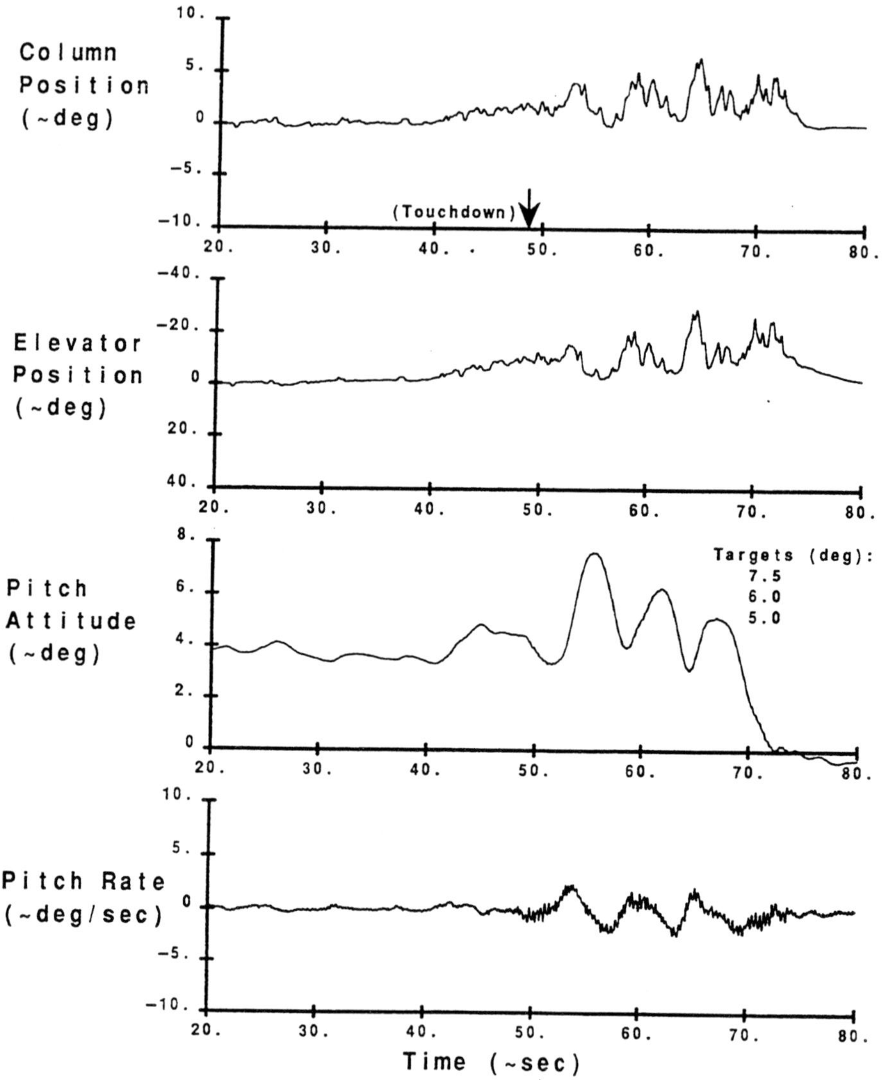

FIGURE 2-13 Time history for 777 attitude tracking on runway, revised control law. Source: McWha.[47]

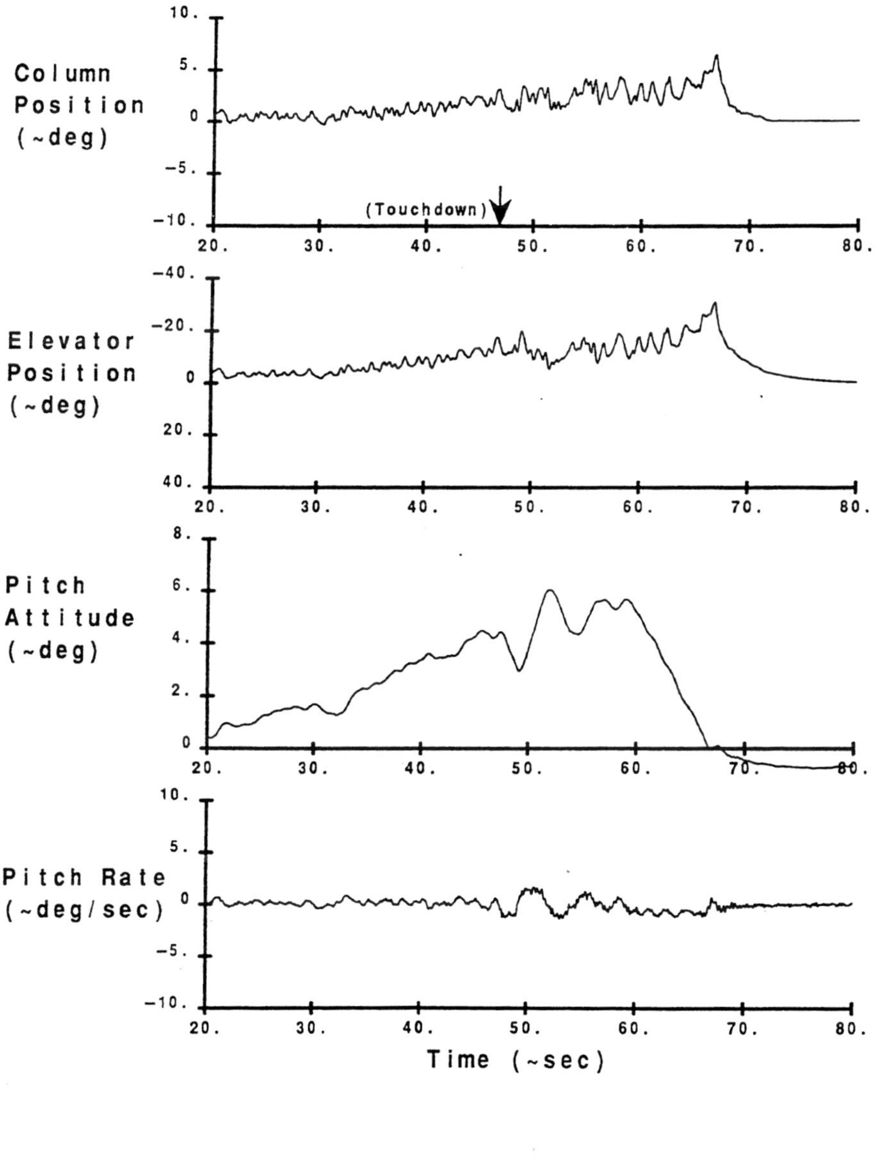

FIGURE 2-14 Time history for 777 attitude tracking on runway, revised control law plus command filter. Source: McWha.[47]

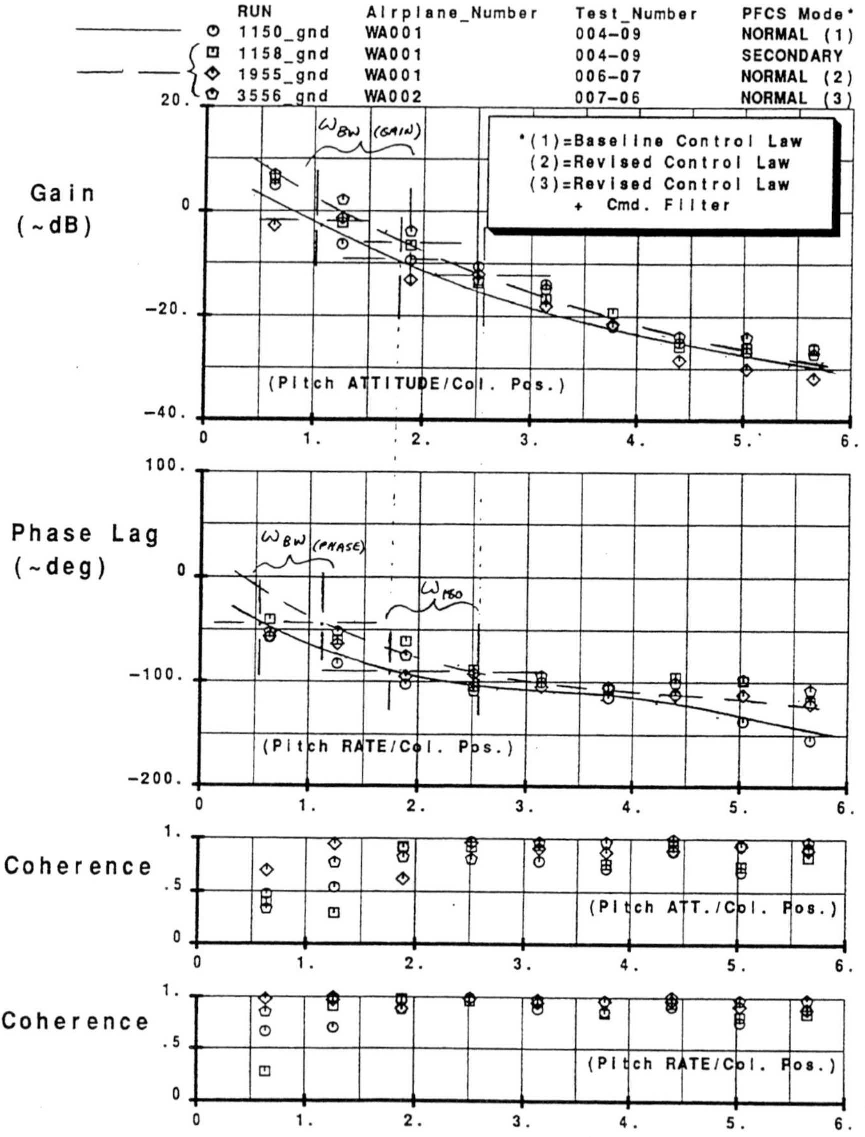

FIGURE 2-15 Bandwidth criteria applied to landing derotation, effect of 777 control law changes on pitch attitude/column position frequency response. Source: McWha.[47]

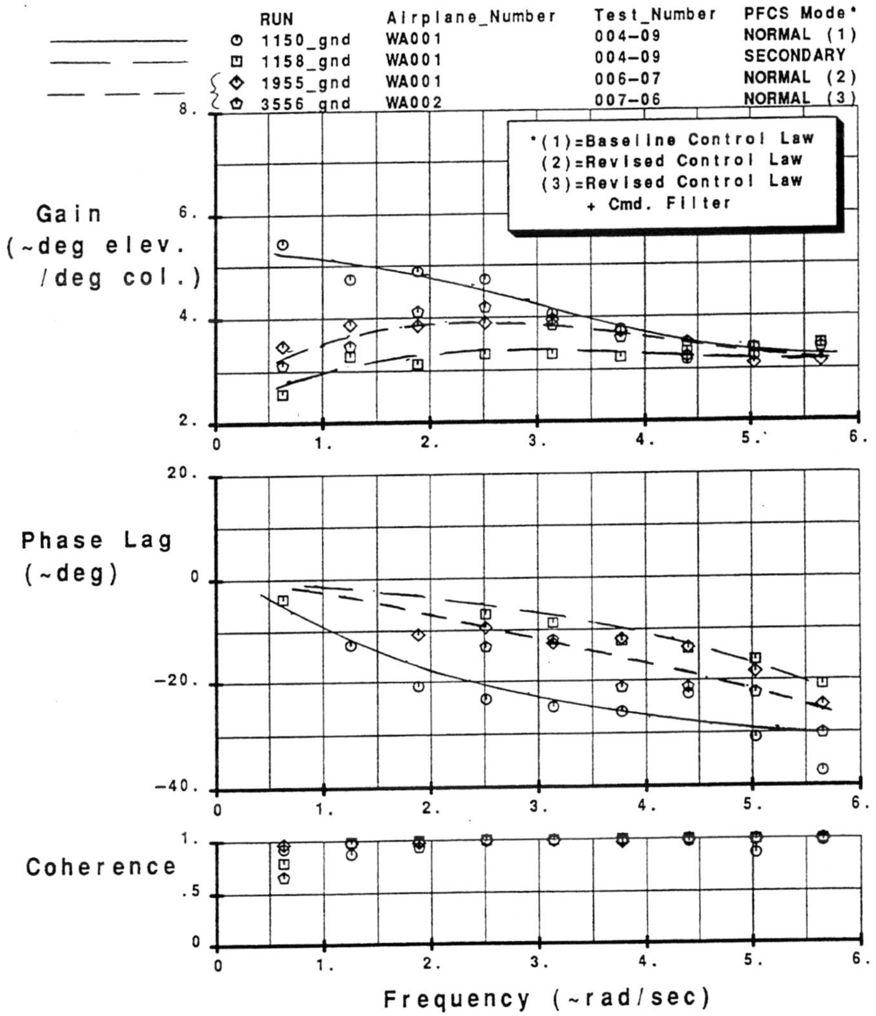

FIGURE 2-16 Elevator/column gain and phase, effect of 777 control law changes on landing derotation. Source: McWha.[47]

Conclusions

The incident described above was a classic Category II PIO, with large-amplitude pilot inputs and both rate- and position-limited elevator activity (as indicated by curve 2 of Figure 2-9). Because of the air-to-ground transition aspects of these incidents (involving airplane, control laws, and pilot), a case could also be made that this was a Category III event.

Landing and derotation is a time of high pilot urgency and gain. For this reason it was assumed during control law development that fixed-base piloted simulations would not be adequate for realistic evaluation in this regime. One lesson from this event is that pilot urgency can be replaced to a significant extent by artificially boosting pilot gain via a suitable tight-tracking task. For example, on-runway attitude tracking showed clear trends in the time history and associated frequency response data. Derotation is a key flight phase and deserves special attention in preflight evaluation. The 777 simulator had the same characteristic as the airplane but was not evaluated as effectively prior to flight test. Also, none of the first five flight test pilots experienced any difficulty during landing, thus illustrating the need for carefully designed flight tests by as many different pilots as possible.

Case 3. McDonnell-Douglas C-17

The C-17 is a four-engine military transport aircraft with a quadruply redundant FBW control system. The aircraft can deliver cargo to austere airfields and land on unpaved runways.

Description of Event

On June 22, 1993, during mission number 176 of the C-17 flight test program, test aircraft T1 experienced a lateral APC event. The test was an approach to landing with hydraulic system #2 inoperative. On final approach, as the pilot corrected for crosswinds using rudders (at about 2 seconds, curve 2, Figure 2-17), he experienced a wing rock. The pilot initiated a lateral command to correct for the wing rock and entered a cycle of oscillatory lateral commands (3 to 12 seconds, curve 1, Figure 2-17). When the aircraft neared 10 degrees of roll attitude, right wing down (at about 8 seconds, curve 1, Figure 2-18) at approximately 15 feet from the ground (curve 3, Figure 2-18) the co-pilot initiated corrective action and attempted commands opposite to the pilot for two cycles (curve 1, Figure 2-17). The aircraft was finally stabilized and a go-around was initiated.

The APC frequency (pilot) was about 0.5 Hz (3.14 rad/Hz) (curve 1, Figure 2-17). During this event, the maximum aileron command was +26 degrees/–39 degrees, as was the actual maximum position of the right aileron (curves 3 and 4, Figure 2-17). The ailerons were rate limited at ±37 degrees/sec (curves 3 and 4, Figure 2-17). Maximum roll attitudes were +10 degrees/–6 degrees (curve 1, Figure 2-18), and maximum roll rates were +14 degrees/sec /–16 degrees/sec (curve 2, Figure 2-18).

Analysis

Analysis showed that the APC event was caused by rate limiting of the ailerons. The rate limiting was caused by overcommanding the surfaces. The overcommand was caused by high gains on both the pilot command path and the feedback paths.

Corrective Action

The total lateral loop gain was reduced, thereby reducing the magnitude of aileron commands for the same stick movement. The overall phase lag of the system was also reduced by optimizing the existing structural filters and removing unnecessary filtering. The use of ailerons was reduced by using spoilers for manual commands only and continuing the use of ailerons for both commands and automated stability augmentation.

Case 4. Airbus A 320

The Airbus A 320 is a twin-engine narrow-body commercial transport with a typical seating capacity of 150. The A 320 entered service in 1988, and approximately 560 A 320s and A 321s are currently in service. (The A 321 is a stretched version of the A 320.)

Description of Event

On April 27, 1995, at about 5:30 p.m. local time, an Airbus A 320 operated by Northwest Airlines was approaching runway 18 at Washington National Airport. Winds were from 220 degrees at 17 knots, gusting to 25 knots. At an altitude of 140 feet, the airplane began a series of roll oscillations that persisted for 30 seconds, reaching a maximum roll of about ±15 degrees (see Figure 2-19, curve 1). Approximately 12 seconds after the start of the roll oscillations, at an altitude of less than 50 feet, the crew initiated a missed approach procedure. The aircraft subsequently made a successful landing. No injuries were reported, and the aircraft was not damaged.

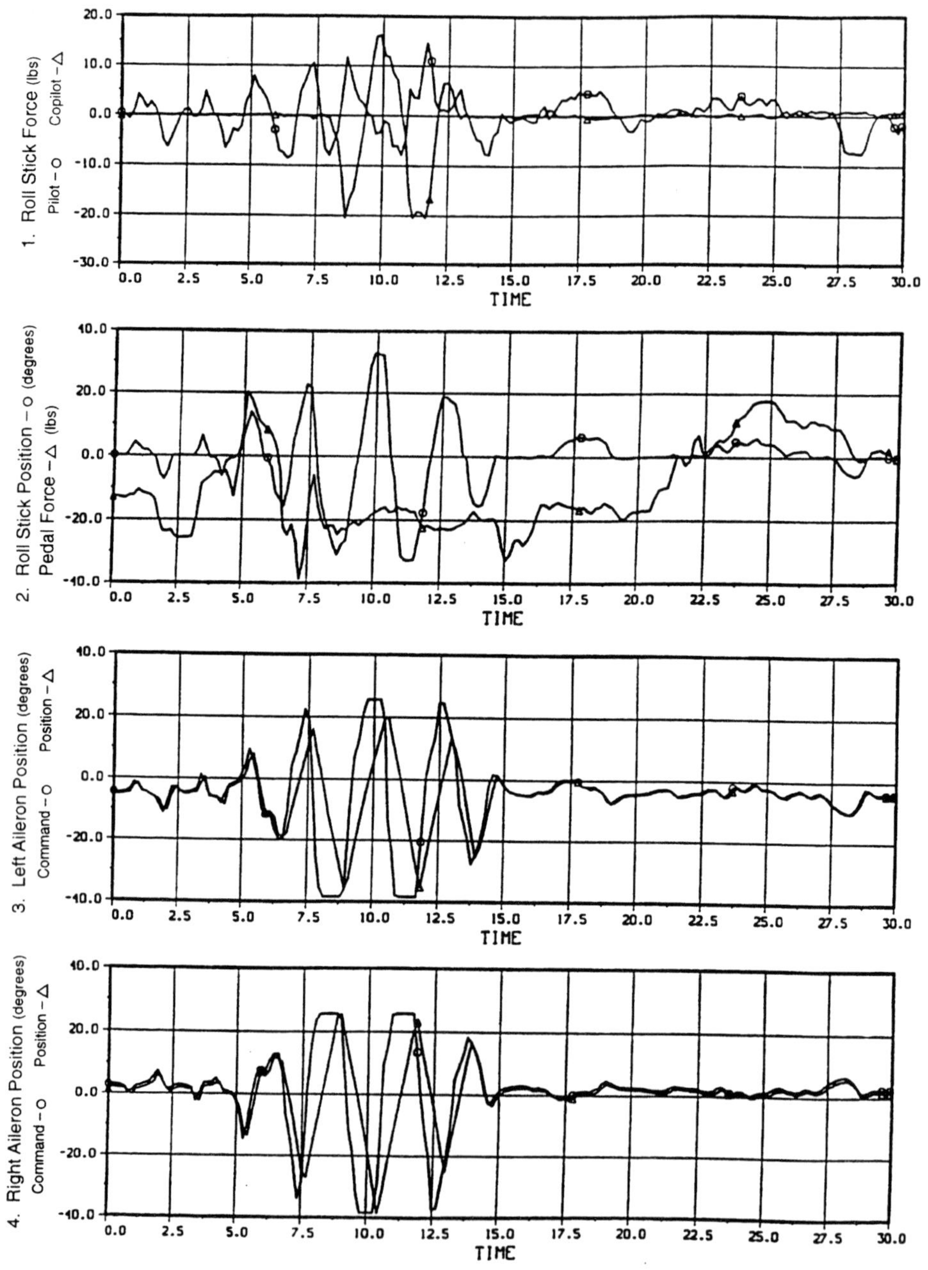

FIGURE 2-17 C-17 test aircraft lateral oscillations during approach to landing with hydraulic system #2 inoperative. Source: Kendall.[38]

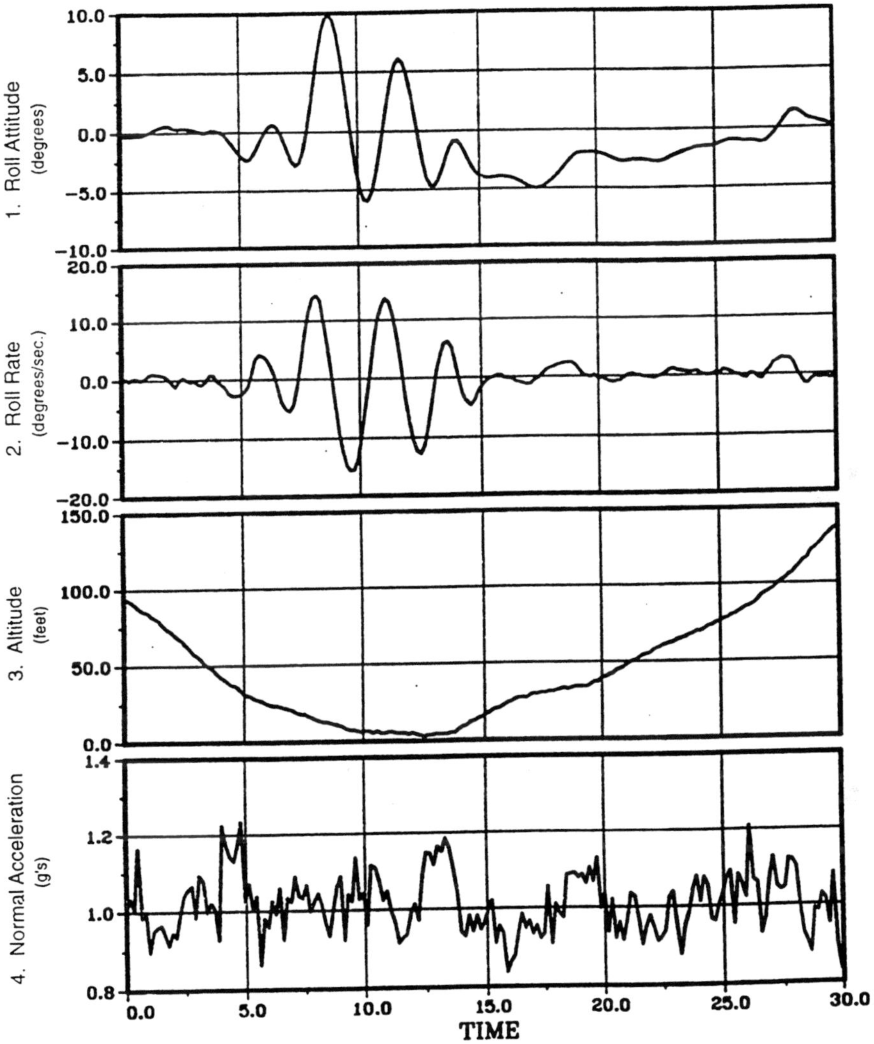

FIGURE 2-18 C-17 test aircraft lateral oscillations during approach to landing with hydraulic system #2 inoperative, continued. Source: Kendall.[38]

As this is an operational airplane, the flight data presented in Figure 2-19 suffer from sampling limitations associated with the data recorder. However, the approximate estimates that can be made indicate the following:

- The PIO frequency was approximately 0.31 Hz (2.5 rad/sec).
- The ailerons achieved maximum deflection of approximately +24 degrees/-20 degrees, and they achieved maximum deflection rates of 35 to 40 degrees/sec.
- The aircraft experienced maximum rolls of approximately +15 degrees (right wing down) and -16 degrees (left wing down). (The National Transportation Safety Board [NTSB] reported a maximum roll of +12.3 degrees/-15.3 degrees.)
- The aircraft experienced maximum roll rates of +23 and -24 degrees/sec.
- During the maximum rolls, the phase difference between stick position (in roll) and aileron position was approximately 216 degrees.
- During the maximum rolls, the phase difference between aileron position and roll was approximately 144 degrees.

Analysis

Data from the flight data recorder (FDR) indicate that, after performing the final turn to align with the runway, the captain made a series of 12 large, rapid, cyclic deflections on his sidestick controller. Most of the deflections were to the maximum values allowed by the mechanical stops on the controller (±20 degrees) (see Figure 2-19, curve 2). Although the pilot had reported experiencing an uncommanded roll of 30 degrees, data from the FDR indicated that aircraft control surfaces operated normally. The NTSB subsequently concluded that this incident was consistent with a PIO and that it was not the result of an uncommanded roll.[52]

During the approach, the flaps were deflected to the 20-degree position, (which is referred to as the CONF 3 position) as part of a noise abatement procedure. Prior to this incident, there had been approximately 10 similar incidents involving other A 320s. In each case, aircraft were landing in gusty wind conditions with flaps in CONF 3, and some pilots experienced difficulty maintaining lateral control. Airbus initially responded to these incidents by issuing a temporary revision to its flight crew operating manual recommending that flaps be set at full deflection (35 degrees, which is referred to as CONF FULL) whenever possible during turbulent landing conditions, to reduce the workload when flying manually. Airbus then developed a flight control software modification to improve the PIO characteristics of the A 320 in CONF 3. This modification reduced the sensitivity of the aircraft to lateral sidestick inputs.

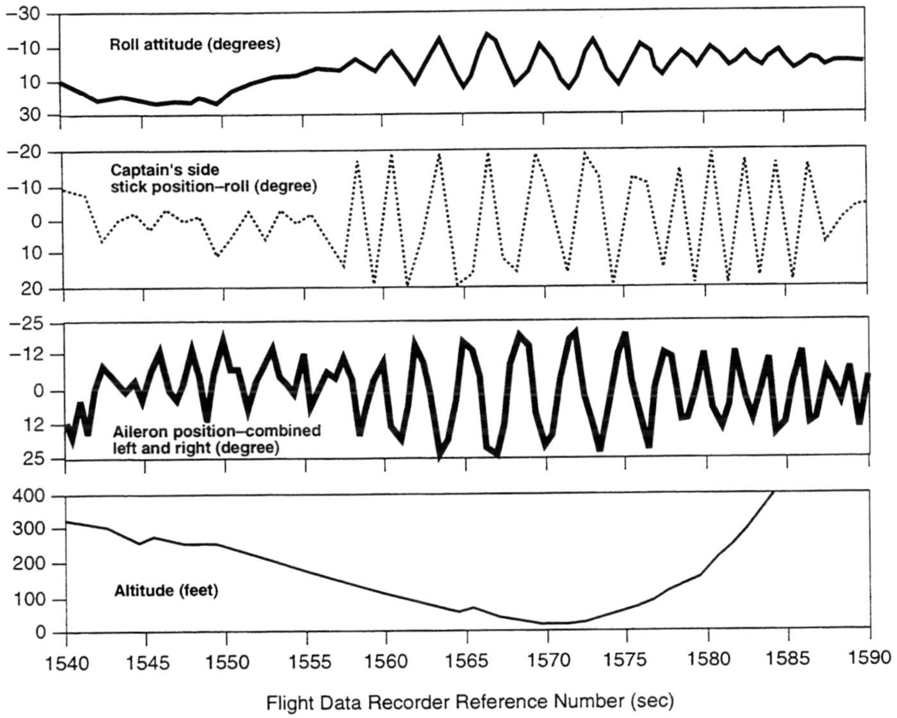

FIGURE 2-19 A 320 incident time history. Source: NTSB.[51]

Although the Airbus service bulletin did not clearly indicate that the modification made important improvements in the handling qualities of the A 320 in CONF 3, Airbus promulgated the information widely. However, neither the French certificating authority (Direction Generale de l'Aviation Civile) nor the FAA made it mandatory. As a result, various A 320 operators handled the matter differently. Some airlines, especially European airlines, disseminated the recommendations and incorporated the modification. Others, including Northwest Airlines, did not. Consequently the aircraft involved in this incident had not been modified, and the pilots were unaware of the Airbus recommendation to use CONF FULL rather than CONF 3 in turbulent conditions. After the event, Northwest Airlines voluntarily installed the modification on all of its A 320s, and subsequently installation of the modification was made mandatory. Operators have reported no problems since incorporating these changes.

Conclusions

Although this problem was corrected by procedural changes and software modifications, the committee concludes that this PIO was probably associated with the lateral flying qualities of the A 320 with flaps in the CONF 3 position. It was probably triggered by a wind gust as the pilot was completing his final turn prior to landing. This incident illustrates that information on APC problems (and solutions) is not always effectively disseminated to the pilots who need it. In fact, incidents such as this one that do not involve injuries or equipment damage often escape scrutiny by government agencies. As a result, unless there are multiple incidents or a serious accident occurs, relevant issues may not be fully resolved.

Case 5. Special Considerations for Rotorcraft

Rotorcraft (i.e., helicopters and tilt rotors such as the V-22 Osprey) have several characteristics that make them prone to PIO:

- limited stability
- significant delays in control effectors because of the time required for rotor response (typically 70 msec) and power actuation (20 to 30 msec)
- coupling of rigid body modes with rotor and transmission modes
- significant inherent cross-coupling of control that is highly nonlinear
- potential coupling with external slung loads

FBW technology has only recently been incorporated into rotorcraft (e.g., V-22, RAH-66 Comanche, and NH-90). Thus, there has been relatively little opportunity to encounter FBW-related PIOs in rotorcraft. However, experience with research helicopters, which is described below, shows that there is reason for caution if not concern.

FBW on rotorcraft can add delays to the FCS response time because of stick filtering and control law computation. For example, one FBW technology demonstrator aircraft (the Advanced Digital Optical Control System, ADOCS) exhibited PIOs in several high gain tasks, including vertical landing, dart-quickstop, and slope landing. End-to-end delays occurred as shown in Figure 2-20. A time history for a landing task is shown in Figure 2-21.[67]

A second example demonstrating the potential for rotorcraft PIOs occurred in an in-flight simulator.[7] The command model was attitude command for pitch and roll; the yaw axis had heading hold. The pilot's inceptors consisted of a spring-loaded force feel system with very little damping, linear stick forces, and relatively low breakout forces.

Another test used a lateral-position tracking task. A hover board mounted on a target vehicle was used to guide the helicopter into a hover over a given point at a given altitude (Figure 2-22). The lateral hover tolerance was ±3 m,

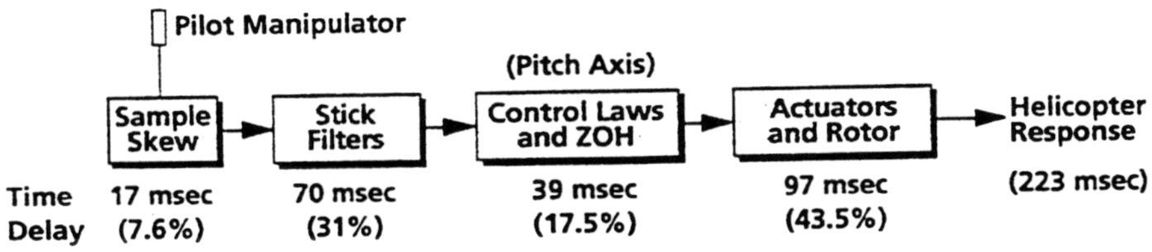

FIGURE 2-20 Response time analysis for the advanced digital optical control system demonstrator. Source: Hamel.[30]

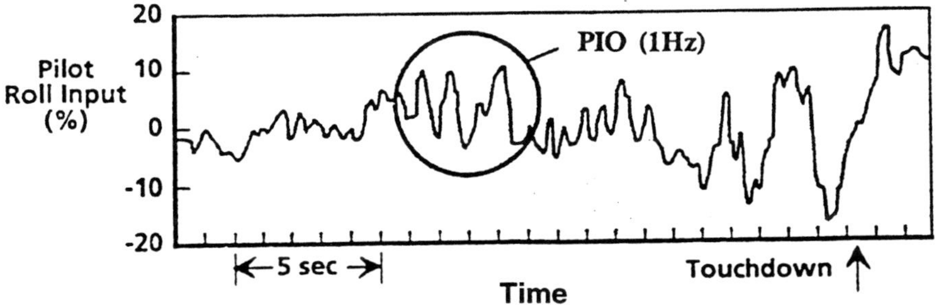

FIGURE 2-21 Sample time history for a rotorcraft vertical landing task. Source: Hamel.[30]

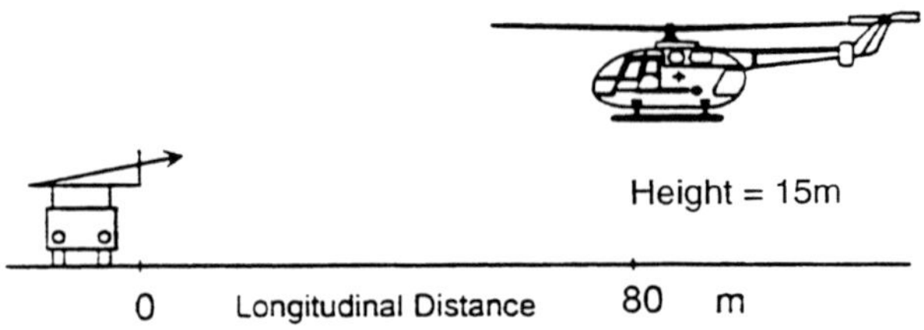

FIGURE 2-22 Schematic drawing of a helicopter tracking a vehicle-mounted hover board. Source: Ockier.[56]

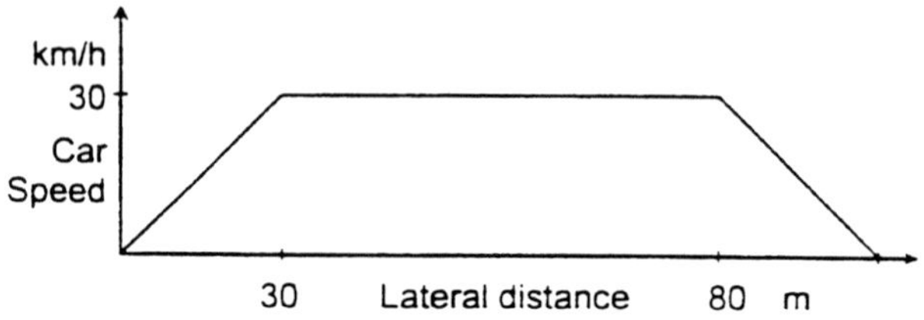

FIGURE 2-23 Helicopter lateral-position tracking task, velocity profile for the lateral vehicle displacement. Ockier.[56]

and the horizontal tolerance was ± 1.5 m. The task was to maintain the hover position relative to the hover board while the target vehicle moved a distance of 100 m in 20 seconds using the velocity pattern shown in Figure 2-23. At the end of the maneuver, a stabilized hover was to be regained.

Figure 2-24 shows the lateral stick input and the bank angle response for the lateral-position tracking task. With no time delay added to the inherent helicopter dynamics (τ = 90 msec), the attitude command model gave a bandwidth of 2.6 rad/sec and a phase delay of 0.1 sec. Although the response is not free of oscillations, there is no PIO tendency and the task was rated as having a CH PR (Cooper-Harper Pilot Rating)* of 5.

Figure 2-25 shows the lateral stick input and bank angle for the same attitude command model with an added time delay of 100 msec (so that τ = 190 msec), resulting in a bandwidth of 2.2 rad/sec and a phase delay of 0.17 sec. A very clear PIO tendency can now be recognized, and the configuration was rated as having a CH PR of 7. Although the time delay is a partial reason for the PIO, there may also be a more important contributor—the biomechanical coupling between aircraft and stick/pilot.

Figure 2-26 shows the two command systems versus the ADS-33D requirement for hover and low speed aggressive maneuvering.[68] The second (PIO-prone) configuration is incorrectly predicted to have Level 2 handling qualities ("adequate to accomplish the mission flight phase, but some increase

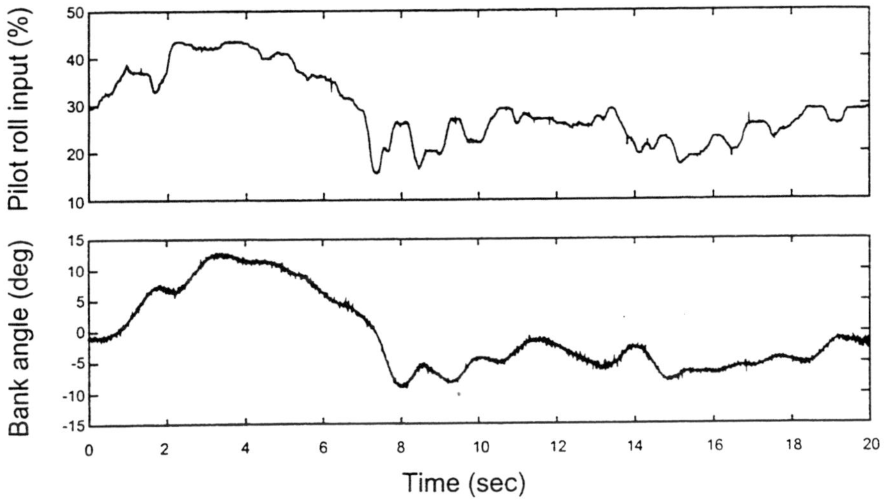

FIGURE 2-24 Time history of the helicopter lateral-position tracking task with no added time delay. Source: Ockier.[56]

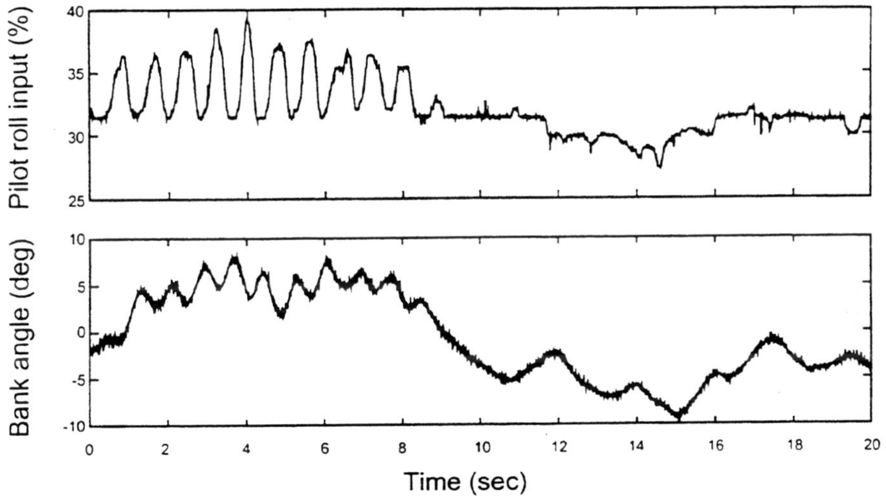

FIGURE 2-25 Time history of the helicopter lateral-position tracking task with 100 msec of added time delay. Source: Ockier.[56]

in pilot workload . . . exists"[71]). This discrepancy underlines the fact that other effects, such as the (biomechanical) aircraft-stick/pilot coupling may have an impact on the introduction of this particular PIO. Such effects are not included in any of the current criteria and would certainly be difficult to predict. It also

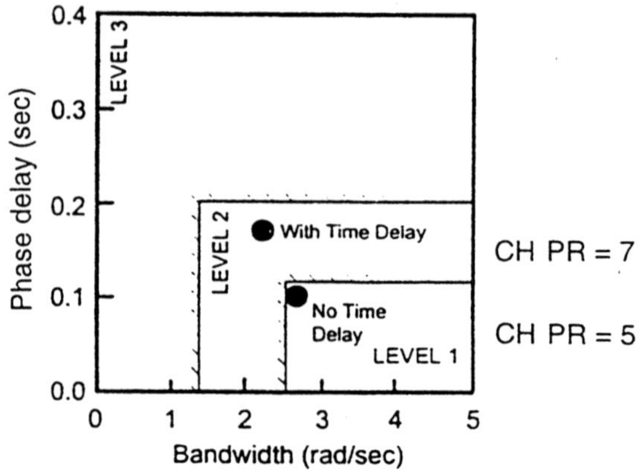

FIGURE 2-26 Small-amplitude handling qualities criterion (target acquisition and tracking) from ADS-33D. Source: Ockier.[56]

illustrates the importance of appropriate force-feel systems for helicopter handling qualities and for the onset of PIOs. For helicopters flying with an attitude command system, additional damping, rapid follow-up trim, or even active, non-linear controllers may be necessary.[56]

A comprehensive review of rotorcraft-pilot coupling potential and experience, including the two cases outlined above, has recently been published.[30]

3

Aircraft-Pilot Coupling as a Current Problem in Aviation

As one aspect of the charge to evaluate the current state of knowledge about adverse APC, the committee was asked to "review and assess recent incidents and accidents in which adverse APC is known or suspected." For several reasons, this has not been a straightforward task for all stages of aviation, and unequivocal answers have been hard to find. For developmental aircraft, the use of elaborate flight test data recorders usually ensures that APC events become a matter of record. Plausible causes can usually be determined and corrective action taken. However, there are no requirements to actively seek out adverse APC tendencies during the development or certification process for either military or commercial aircraft. Thus, an aircraft being developed might not be exposed to PIO-prone situations.

Once an aircraft enters operational service, multichannel, high, fidelity high sample-rate flight-data recording equipment is no longer used to monitor flight performance. The FDRs installed in commercial transports have far less capability, and military aircraft may have none at all. Other factors that work against a concrete and unequivocal assessment of APC potential are discussed below. In an effort to address the task of reviewing and assessing recent incidents and accidents, the committee examined, more extensively than anticipated, a variety of information sources, including accident and incident investigations, flight data recordings, and pilots. The principal sources of information are discussed in separate sections of this chapter.

TRENDS FROM A REVIEW OF ACCIDENTS AND INCIDENTS

To review and assess recent incidents and accidents, the committee approached the problem over a broad front. This review was the focus of two workshops held to gather the best information available (see Appendix C for participants). To supplement the workshop data, subgroups of the committee examined numerous potentially relevant databases, held lengthy discussions with a Russian colleague, and went to Europe to collect information available there. The following partial list indicates the scope of the sources examined:

- NTSB reports
- Aviation Safety Reporting System data (1990–1994)
- technical literature
- briefings by representatives of several airlines
- information in the public domain (e.g., articles in Aviation Week and Space Technology and information on the Internet)
- workshop briefings by parties involved in specific APC events
- workshop briefings by specialists from the U.S. Air Force Wright Laboratory and research contractors
- internal FAA incident data
- briefings by the Air Accidents Investigation Branch of the United Kingdom
- developmental experience from aircraft companies (Boeing, McDonnell Douglas, Lockheed Martin, British Aerospace, Airbus, and Saab)
- manufacturer safety publications
- U.S. military flight test experience

After an extensive investigation and review, the committee was able to identify five features or trends of APC-related accidents.

1. APC events almost always occur during the development of new classes of aircraft that operate in new flight regimes or employ new technologies, such as FBW. This is also apparent in Tables 1-1 and 1-2, which summarize adverse APC events of varying severity in the development of advanced aircraft, including almost all partial or total FBW aircraft for which data were available. These include high performance military aircraft, such as the F-16, Tornado, F-18, YF-22, and JAS 39; large bomber and transport aircraft, such as the B-2, A 320, C-17, and Boeing 777; and the Space Shuttle Orbiter.
2. Even during development testing, PIOs and APC events are rare. Many pilots conduct extensive flight test operations with no difficulties until just the right combination of triggering event, pilot dynamics, and effective aircraft dynamics occurs.

3. Once an APC event is discovered in the development stage, it becomes highly visible. Developers are motivated to uncover the sources and contributing factors and to correct deficiencies. In other words, APC susceptibility is often detected and corrected as a natural part of the development, flight testing, and certification process.
4. Confirmed occurrences of APC-related incidents on operational FBW aircraft are rare, although some exist.
5. Analysis of severe PIOs almost always show that control surfaces were rate limited during the event. (Rate limiting is indicated when a graph of control surface position versus time produces a triangular plot, as in curve 5 of Figure 2-7 and curve 2 of Figure 2-9).

The contrast between the presence of PIOs and other APC events in nearly all FBW aircraft during development tests by highly skilled, focused test pilots and the near absence of APC events in operational stages with line pilots has been noted as a "curious disconnect." This disconnect can, perhaps, be interpreted in two ways, both of them speculative. First, all major PIO tendencies have been discovered in the course of development. This explanation is most applicable if the development process includes a dedicated, effective effort to discover the circumstances (e.g., maneuvers and aircraft and FCS configurations) in which APC-prone tendencies are the most severe (for instance, when processes such as those recommended in Chapter 4 are applied). For some aircraft, however, an active investigation of APC characteristics may not have been conducted throughout the development process (or the effort to discover APC problems may have been flawed). Although these aircraft may appear to be immune to PIOs, it may simply be that they did not happen to encounter the conditions that would lead to a PIO with that particular aircraft. If that is the case, an unexpected PIO could result when production aircraft do encounter the necessary conditions. Unanticipated APC events usually greatly focus the attention of the responsible engineers and make them true believers in the potential hazards associated with APC events.

A second interpretation of why some operational aircraft have no reports of PIOs or other APC events is that there has been a detection or reporting oversight. This could be because of differences between test pilots and line pilots, who may not have an adequate understanding of PIOs or who may interpret APC events as signs of pilot error. Such factors could lead to nonreporting of PIOs that occur in operational aircraft. Flight safety demands that operational pilots avoid PIOs and other difficult situations rather than seek them out. Other reasons for the absence of reported incidents may be that accident investigators do not adequately consider the extent to which APC events contribute to incidents or accidents, and there may be inadequacies in recording capabilities and/or analytical procedures.

In any event, the committee was not able to assess fully the existing exposure of APC in operational fleets because of limitations in the reporting systems. Most currently available FDR systems do not sample at rates sufficient to allow investigation of high-frequency, oscillatory APC events. Older FDRs do not sample enough of the relevant parameters to identify potential APC phenomena. Requirements for improved FDRs are being considered that would increase the likelihood of identifying APC tendencies before catastrophic events occur. However, the temporal resolution of improved FDRs may still not be sufficient to identify high-frequency APC events.

Reporting of APC events by pilots to safety reporting systems, such as the Aviation Safety Reporting System, is also thought to be limited by cultural factors. Because there has been a historical association of PIOs with inexperience and poor airmanship, pilots are often reluctant to admit having been involved in a PIO or APC event. This problem is exacerbated by the lack of a clear boundary between a benign APC event (e.g., an oscillation experienced by a novice student or a turbulence-induced oscillation) and an adverse APC event that could result in catastrophe.

FLIGHT DATA RECORDERS

Depending upon the sophistication of the FDRs and the number of parameters being recorded, FDRs make possible accurate reconstruction of events associated with a particular flight. The first requirement for installing FDRs on commercial aircraft was issued by the Civil Aeronautics Administration, the predecessor to the FAA, on August 1, 1958. Similar requirements were subsequently issued by regulatory authorities in other nations. To facilitate investigations of serious incidents and accidents, crashworthy FDRs are now required on most commercial aircraft in airline service.

The number of parameters that the U.S. Federal Aviation Regulations require crashworthy FDRs to measure on a particular aircraft varies from 6 to 34, depending upon the aircraft's date of manufacture and the date the FAA issued the type certification for that aircraft. Older FDRs only collect basic flight data: altitude, airspeed, heading, normal "g," microphone keying, and time. Newer FDRs also collect data such as pitch attitude, roll attitude, and either control-surface positions or control-column positions. Data sampling rates are generally once per second, although a few parameters are recorded at higher rates, eight per second being the highest. Current regulations allow some aircraft equipped with the old six-channel recorders to use them into the twenty-first century. However, a proposed change to the Federal Aviation Regulations would increase the number of monitored parameters on new aircraft to 88, including a requirement to monitor parameters such as cockpit flight-control input forces. Nevertheless, the proposed sampling rates would be similar to the ones now required of older recorders.

In addition to FDRs, other recorders are also available, and many individual operators have installed them voluntarily in their aircraft. These recorders, known as quick access recorders (QARs), are usually not crashworthy, but they record many additional parameters besides the ones required by FAA regulations. For example, some QARs can record as many as 400 separate parameters. In addition, the high capacity memories of QARs means they can store data for many more flight hours than FDRs, and the data are stored on easily removable media, such as optical disks. Most QARs record data at the same rates as FDRs required by regulation. QARs are generally used to monitor the performance of aircraft and engine systems for operational and maintenance purposes. They can also be used to evaluate crew actions and performance.

FLIGHT OPERATIONAL QUALITY ASSURANCE

Regular examination of FDR or QAR data can also be used to identify potential problems affecting flight safety. Such efforts, which are known in U.S. industry as Flight Operational Quality Assurance (FOQA) programs, may reveal adverse trends before they result in an accident or serious incident. FOQA programs use ground-based computers to analyze QAR data to verify that aircraft systems are operating normally, that aircraft are being operated in accordance with standard operating procedures, and that they are being flown within the safe flight envelope.*

Airlines in many parts of the world outside the United States, especially in Europe, have had FOQA programs for many years. However, this has not been the normal practice in the United States. British Airways, which has been a leading proponent of FOQA programs, claims that its FOQA program has identified potential causes of accidents, which were then eliminated through appropriate corrective action.

Modern FDRs and QARs have the potential to facilitate the investigation of APC-related accidents and incidents by allowing investigators to compare many relevant parameters, including pilot control-surface inputs, FCS command signals transmitted to control-surface actuators, control-surface position, and aircraft motion. In fact, Airbus has recommended using a FOQA process to search specifically for APC phenomena during routine operations. Safety analysis equipment would need to be programmed and personnel trained to detect specific traits; a FOQA program would also provide quantitative data on how frequently APC-related phenomena might occur during the routine operation of conventional and FBW commercial aircraft. However, it would be necessary to increase the data sampling rates of certain parameters because the current rates are too low to allow satisfactory APC or PIO analysis. Generally, rate adjustments can be made by changes in software, but the possibilities may be limited by the design of recorders and their interfaces with particular aircraft. Depending upon the limitations, the costs could be quite high for an entire fleet. Proper searches for and examination of PIO phenomena would require a sampling rate for some parameters of at least 10 per second.

Analysis of flight data from commercial aircraft on a routine basis in the United States has been limited by several factors. Airline pilots have been concerned about possible punitive actions by management or regulatory agencies in the event that FOQA programs reveal cockpit crew errors. Airlines themselves have been concerned about enforcement penalties that might be imposed by the FAA if operational violations are identified. And the aviation industry in general has been concerned about adverse consequences if news organizations or plaintiffs' lawyers were able to use the Freedom of Information Act to access FOQA data supplied to the FAA in confidence for the purpose of improving safety. Several major U.S. airlines are now cautiously initiating FOQA programs, but these are based on individual agreements between unions and management. They also depend on assurances of the FAA administrator that information revealed for the purposes of improving flight safety will not be used in a punitive way. Proposals for FAA regulations granting similar protections are also being drafted.

Industry safety experts and organizations like the Flight Safety Foundation have long advocated the need for comprehensive, nonpunitive FOQA reporting systems. The potential benefits are obvious, and removing the threat of punitive action would significantly increase support for FOQA programs.

MILITARY AIRCRAFT

Although many military aircraft are fitted with various types of recorders, including (in some cases) crash survivable FDRs, the U.S. military has often been reluctant to require crash-survivable FDRs, even on military versions of commercial aircraft where recording capability is readily available. The investigation of the YF-22 accident, which is discussed in Chapter 2, indicated that investigators would have had a much more difficult time identifying the details of the APC event without the sophisticated data recording system that was installed on this developmental aircraft.

The death of the Secretary of Commerce in 1996 in the crash of a military transport has led to additional emphasis on the installation of crash-survivable FDRs on some military aircraft; however, that will not address the problem of adequately investigating APC-related aspects of crashes involving operational combat aircraft.

ACCIDENT INVESTIGATIONS

In the past, PIO phenomena have not generally been recognized as a potential cause of accidents involving commercial aircraft in service. Although the data collected by FDRs on commercial aircraft have been adequate to identify flight path oscillations, for the most part these data have not been adequate to determine definitively if APC caused the oscillations or if the accidents involved APC phenomena.

Most new FBW commercial aircraft have experienced one or more APC events during development, some of them severe. The sophisticated flight test instrumentation fitted to development aircraft enabled those APC events to be identified and the problems eliminated before the aircraft was put into operation. Once in service, however, the aircraft FDRs and QARs can not detect PIO problems, except in the most fortuitous circumstances. Therefore, investigations of commercial accidents seldom mention PIO as a contributory factor.

Nevertheless there may have been a few APC-related incidents in operational service. Airbus, which has more than 700 FBW aircraft in airline operation, has more FBW experience than any other manufacturer. In all the flight hours accumulated by this fleet to date, 10 possible PIO incidents have been identified. Although Airbus acknowledges only three as genuine PIOs, the problems associated with these 10 incidents have been identified and fixed. One of them is described in case study 4 (Chapter 2).

Because APC events may appear in operational service, improvements in the capabilities of FDRs and QARs will make it easier for investigators to determine the extent to which APC phenomena are present in specific incidents and accidents, provided recorder sampling rates are adequate. Therefore, the ability to detect APC problems could be enhanced by educating reviewers of FOQA programs, as well as accident investigators, regarding the existence of APC hazards and how to identify them.

4

Precluding Adverse Aircraft-Pilot Coupling Events

INTRODUCTION

Current requirements and processes employed during the development of military and commercial aircraft do not preclude adverse APC events or ensure that they will be recognized when they do occur. APC-related incidents and accidents have occurred in both developmental and operational (nondevelopmental) aircraft. A study of those events has identified some lessons and some analyses and tests that could significantly reduce the risk of APC events. This chapter outlines a structured approach to the development of FCSs that should minimize the potential for adverse APC events in flight.

LESSONS LEARNED

The committee believes that flight experience with conventional and FBW FCSs substantiates the following lessons with regard to APC events:

- Truly optimizing aircraft handling qualities, by definition, reduces susceptibility to APC problems (because an aircraft with APC problems cannot be considered to have optimized handling qualities).
- Attempts to optimize aircraft handling qualities have sometimes inadvertently led to APC problems that were not recognized until after the fact.

- Structural dynamics may significantly influence closed-loop control systems and must be considered in the design process, particularly for large aircraft.
- The FCS must accommodate transitions between different modes in a way that is consistent with the pilot's expectations. When many modes are necessary to meet performance-related requirements, the resulting increase in system complexity can complicate system development and validation.
- Transitions between modes, especially in the case of failures, can cause unexpected transients that may trigger APC events. Therefore, automatic step changes in surface commands should be carefully analyzed in the FCS design.
- APC problems have occurred during development because of the improper or incomplete allocation of system parameters (e.g., system time delays) among subsystems.
- APC problems have occasionally occurred because APC criteria were not periodically revisited as the design proceeded.
- Simulation and flight testing should include thorough evaluations of high-gain, task-oriented flying qualities specifically to test for APC characteristics.
- Sequences of "carefree flight"* during simulation and early flight testing when pilots actively search for APC possibilities are essential.
- A number of pilots should be exposed to simulation and flight tests of new aircraft as early as possible in order to investigate APC characteristics.
- The effects of various combinations of aircraft system modes, failure states, and pilot actions should be evaluated.
- During testing, all anomalous results should be investigated. Sometimes this is not done because of time pressure or inexperience.
- APC susceptibility should be assumed until proven otherwise.
- "A pilot would never do that" is not a valid argument for excluding a particular series of pilot commands from analysis or simulation.

Lessons learned from the committee's review of APC-related incidents and accidents include the following:

- Civil and military organizations, both national and international, approach APC concerns in a variety of ways. Some focus on formal APC criteria, while others rely primarily on empirical methods and rules of thumb based on experience with prior aircraft. On the one hand, the committee found that no approach consistently produced aircraft free of adverse APC characteristics. On the other hand, the committee found that no approach consistently produced aircraft with unacceptable APC characteristics.

- Manufacturers of civil and military aircraft often consider the approaches they use to address adverse APC part of the proprietary design and manufacturing process. The APC characteristics of current aircraft are often treated as proprietary or classified performance data, which tends to inhibit the exchange of APC-related information and interferes with cooperative efforts to eliminate adverse APC.
- In many cases, indications of sensitivity to APC were identified in simulations and analysis, but these indications were dismissed prematurely. At a minimum, potential APC sensitivity should be taken as an early warning that requires further investigation.
- All signals critical to the FCS must be fault tolerant and must be accommodated adequately by reversionary modes.
- Designs should minimize phase delays due to rate saturation (from surface actuators or other sources). In addition, integrator windup must be avoided. (See the section on technical fixes near the end of this chapter.)

RECOMMENDED PROCESSES FOR IDENTIFYING AND PRECLUDING ADVERSE AIRCRAFT-PILOT COUPLING EVENTS

There are opportunities for improving the processes used during the analysis, design, testing, and certification phases of a development program. The committee believes that wider use of the following policies and procedures would reduce the potential for adverse APC events.

Management Policies

Management should recognize that available APC evaluation criteria are tentative and incomplete but will continue to improve as the design of the aircraft and aircraft systems evolves. Management should also recognize that opportunities for adverse APC are often created when new systems are introduced. Therefore, periodic reviews, pilot evaluations, and criteria updates are warranted. Senior management should ensure the continuous implementation of the following general policies:

- APC susceptibility should be assumed; evaluations aimed at minimizing APC risk should be an essential part of vehicle design and development from the beginning of the program and should continue through vehicle certification and entry into service.
- A highly structured systems-engineering approach to APC risk reduction should be implemented. This approach should require all relevant disciplines to be aware of and focus attention on the APC risk

reduction process from early in the program until the aircraft enters service.

- A multidisciplinary team should develop the FCS. This team should include representatives of the following disciplines: piloting, flight controls, stability and control, aerodynamics, structures, avionics, electrical power, human factors, and maintenance.
- Team leaders should be prepared to facilitate the resolution of problems, to convey to higher management the need to investigate thoroughly potential APC problems, and to withstand the pressure to avoid program delays by cutting corners on APC risk reduction.
- The relevant teams should agree early on design and evaluation criteria for flight qualities and APC risk reduction. All team members must be aware of the consequences of adverse APC events and must rigorously apply the selected criteria.
- Team charters should include procedures for resolving differences of opinion regarding steps to be taken to identify and eliminate adverse APC tendencies.

Design Process

The overall design process is illustrated in Figure 4-1. The key steps in the process that focus on the elimination of adverse APC events are discussed below.

Establish Flight Control Philosophy and Objectives

The basic flight control philosophy should incorporate safety, past experience, customer requirements, and company strategies. Different types of aircraft (fighters, transports, etc.) often have significantly different control philosophies. The control philosophy may include the following elements: the aircraft-pilot interface (inceptors, displays, etc.); pilot control authority; augmentation of handling qualities; and enhanced control functions, such as envelope protection. The philosophy should be understood clearly by each member of the team involved in developing focused requirements and objectives for the system.

The type of inceptor can significantly affect the design process and methods of evaluation. For example, there are major differences between a large-displacement center-stick inceptor and a minimal displacement side-stick inceptor. Piloting techniques may differ for different inceptor designs, and the selection of handling qualities and APC criteria may be influenced by the type of inceptor. The type of inceptor may also be important to the simulator and aircraft design teams because the geometry, hardware, type of simulation, etc.,

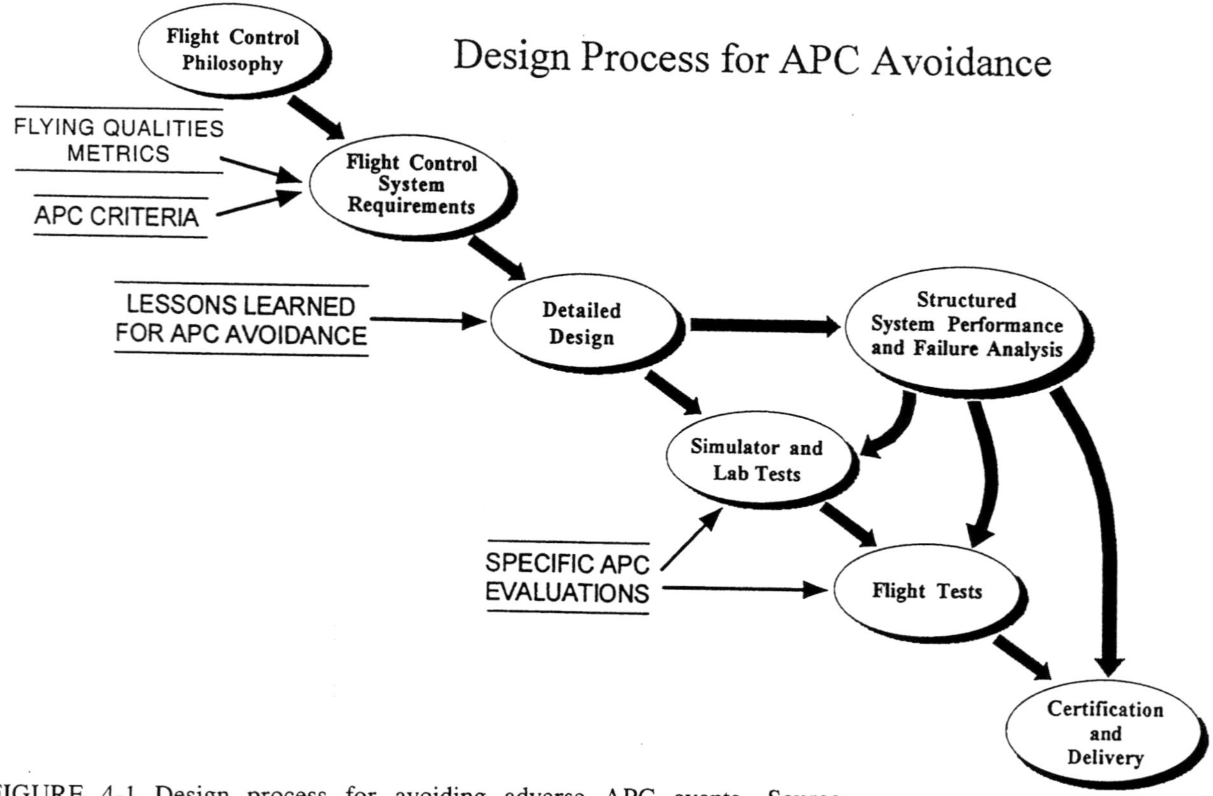

FIGURE 4-1 Design process for avoiding adverse APC events. Source: McWha.[47]

TABLE 4-1 Flying Qualities Requirements and Metrics

Requirement	Key Metrics
Inceptor characteristics (each axis)	Type of inceptor
	Force vs. displacement (static)
	Gradients
	Detent-breakout force
	• Centering
	• Dead zone
	• Hysteresis
	Damping, inertia, bobweight effects, etc.
	Mass balance (pitch)
Maneuvering Characteristics	
General	Control-surface sizing
	Actuator rates and bandwidth
	Trim
	Command linearity (with inceptor position)
Dynamic	Pitch short period and phugoid
	Roll/yaw responses
	Effective time delays
	Control harmony
Steady state	Pitch controller force/g
	Speed stability
	Roll/yaw
	Roll rate/controller command
Mode Transitions	Transition time
	Characteristics across transition
	Minimal transient

are all influenced by the inceptor selection. For all of these reasons, it is important that the design team reach agreement or develop a plan to reach an agreement very early in the design process on the type of inceptor.

Define Flying Qualities Requirements

Good flying qualities are fundamental to the elimination of adverse APC. These are defined in the form of requirements with relevant metrics to be satisfied. Table 4-1 provides an outline of some fundamental qualities that are directly reflected in the aircraft and FCS designs. The design team should select the appropriate metrics (and values) for a specific aircraft that will maximize the overall performance of the aircraft in terms of its ability to execute assigned tasks safely (which implies good flying qualities). Additional criteria and metrics that specifically address APC should be developed and added to this list. Among the additional criteria that should be considered are the following:

- Aircraft-Bandwidth*/Phase Delay, ω_{BW} and τ_p
- Gain/Phase Template, including ω_{180}/Average Phase Rate
- Smith-Geddes Attitude-Dominant Type III
- Neal-Smith
- Dropback

Each of these criteria is described in detail in Chapter 6. These criteria relate primarily to maneuvering characteristics and should not be viewed as pass/fail tests but as ways of alerting the analysis and design teams to potential sources of APC risk. The criteria can be refined for different aircraft types and can increase confidence that APC risk in the design has been minimized.

Not all of the criteria are equally appropriate for all control system designs and aircraft types. For example, Boeing has found that the Smith-Geddes Attitude-Dominant Type III criterion is probably overly conservative when applied to the roll axis of large transport aircraft.[54] The manufacturers of the YF-22 and F-16 have had similar concerns with respect to the control system designs. Even with these limitations, however, design teams should use each available criterion as an indicator and recommend improvements or adjustments when there is sufficient evidence to do so.

The existing control system flying qualities and APC criteria for Category I PIOs appear to work best with FCSs with a "classical" response, and the design team should consider this fact early in the design process. For example, one reason the F-22 program decided to use a classical approach to control system design was to prevent ambiguities between pilot comments on FCS performance and the results of analyses using conventional criteria for the nonclassical YF-22 and F-16 design concepts and approach. If a nonclassical approach is selected, the team should be aware of the ambiguities that may result from the use of conventional criteria.

The APC criteria listed above need to be supplemented to address Category II and III APC phenomena. The committee emphasizes that, when changes are made to the FCS as the development evolves, the new configuration should be reassessed against the APC criteria. Until reliable criteria and analysis tools become available for Category II and III phenomena, reliance must be placed on comprehensive simulation tests and, perhaps, flight tests.

Detailed Flight Control Design

Once flying qualities requirements have been established, they should be integrated with other design requirements that address reliability, availability, and maintainability. A well structured process for developing control laws should be implemented. This is an iterative process requiring extensive communication between the team members and pilots. The lessons learned for APC prevention, which are presented above, should be used to formulate design goals such as the following:

- Ensure that, wherever possible, the control strategy applies to all tasks under all flight conditions.
- Design the system to perform consistently throughout as much of the flight envelope as possible to minimize the chance that the pilot will incorrectly modify his behavior to compensate for system response characteristics.
- Verify that the detailed design is satisfactory in terms of potential problem areas such as integrator windup, the impact of power interrupts, and switching feedback capacitors.
- Minimize the number of modes and failure states, consistent with aircraft performance requirements.
- Ensure smooth transition between modes and failure states.
- Avoid designs that depend on the high end of normally available aircraft performance (e.g., a flight path profile that is only achievable with all engines at full thrust).
- To achieve predictable input-output characteristics, avoid nonlinear design features; design for linear proportional responses whenever possible.
- Include appropriate structural dynamics models.
- Check that the probability of saturating actuator rate and/or position is extremely unlikely under all circumstances, including maximum maneuvering rates and severe turbulence.
- Allow sufficient authority and priority for the augmentation functions during extreme maneuvers.
- Minimize phase delays caused by rate-limiting effects.
- Ensure that time delays are accounted for in development models for simulation and analysis.
- Ensure that key system parameters, such as effective time delays, have been allocated and included in subsystem specifications.
- Analyze the system behavior in great detail to understand the effects of all nonlinearities in the design; analyze what happens when command inputs saturate the control system, especially when the SAS (stability augmentation system) may also be working (or trying to work), which can lead to unrealizable demands on control-surface actuators.

Specifications for all major FCS elements and interfaces, including the flying qualities metrics defined earlier, should be prepared and translated into appropriate parameters. These specifications also should address APC lessons learned.

The availability of critical data significantly influences the design process. The final design of a FCS is dependent on the aerodynamic database that describes the aircraft, the weight and inertia of the aircraft, the rate and hinge-moment capability of the actuation systems, the effectiveness of the control devices, the structural rigidity of the aircraft and control surfaces, the dynamic behavior of the aircraft, etc. Unfortunately, these data are almost never available at the start of the control-system design process; they are progressively released and updated throughout the development process. Often, a new aircraft is flying before all this information is known. The control-system design team must decide how the evolving design data will be incorporated into the design process.

Simulators (both ground and in-flight) are key elements in the design process. Availability, schedule, cost, etc., all require early agreement on how simulators will be used.

The requirements of the FCS may significantly affect the design of other systems. The design team should consider how these requirements can be identified early in the process and should communicate them to other system design teams. An important requirement (particularly from an APC perspective) is the rate capability of the actuation system. The hydraulic or mechanical limitation on the actuator rate is a key factor in the susceptibility to Category II APC. If the aircraft design is finalized with severe rate limitations, problems in designing the control system can be greatly magnified. The integrity, availability, and redundancy of sensors and other subsystems could be a source of triggering events if these parameters are not adequately integrated into the overall design.

Structured Analysis of System Performance

In this phase of the design process, the effects on flying qualities of many factors are assessed in detail. A structured analysis of system performance can provide guidance on where to apply certain requirements and can focus subsequent testing. A matrix of variations should be considered for analyzing the following factors:

- flight conditions
- aircraft configuration
- aircraft loading
- atmospheric conditions
- air/ground states
- FCS modes

- failure states for the FCS and all interfaces
- structural influences

From an APC standpoint, these factors should be assessed in the context of upsets or abuses that may occur in conjunction with large or otherwise inappropriate pilot inputs under high workload conditions.

Simulation Considerations

Simulators and simulator pilots play a significant role in developing the FCS and reducing the risk of adverse APC. In the selection of the simulation approach, a number of factors should be considered.

- Installing the correct pilot inceptors is critical. It is very difficult to extrapolate handling qualities and APC characteristics between different types of inceptors.
- The end-to-end time delays in the simulation must be understood, and any differences between the simulated and real systems should be minimized. The simulation is always a degradation of the real world, and the effects of this degradation must be considered.
- To minimize the time delay for simulations of handling qualities, the simulator visual scene may have to be restricted.
- Ground-based simulations may not adequately reveal the existence of adverse APC because (1) they lack acceleration cues, (2) the visual systems are less than satisfactory, and (3) it is difficult to instill a sense of urgency in the pilot. Moving-base simulators may be better than fixed-base simulators for testing the PVS in some parts of the flight envelope. However, the committee believes an excellent visual display system is more important than a moving base in most cases because instrument-rated pilots are trained to rely upon visual rather than acceleration cues. (Simulation is addressed more extensively in Chapter 5.)
- In-flight simulations solve many of the problems inherent in ground simulations, but because they are very expensive, in-flight simulations must be well planned and used judiciously.

Simulation, Laboratory, and Flight Test Flying Qualities and Aircraft-Pilot Coupling Evaluations

The committee discovered a strong industry consensus on the importance of selecting simulation tasks for detecting APC tendencies. Adverse tendencies that are evident with low-gain inputs are easily observed and can be eliminated in the design process. However, discovering, minimizing, or eliminating most adverse APC requires high-gain pilot inputs. Thus, the tasks selected for simulator pilots should generate high pilot gain.

The committee believes that a desirable way to generate high gains is to simulate real aircraft tasks that emphasize precision PVS performance because realistic high-gain tasks make problems more credible. However, it is useful to include some tasks that naturally maximize pilot gain but that may not be typical of normal flight operations. These tasks should stress the PVS to its limits, thereby ensuring that it is not susceptible to APC phenomena under even the most extreme conditions. High gain tasks should be repeated several times. A variety of tasks should also be included that focus on possible differences in pilot responses to visual and acceleration cues.

In the absence of applicable APC criteria and analysis tools, the ground simulator is the only convenient place to evaluate the wide range of conditions that could produce hazardous Category III APC events. By definition, Category III APC events are unpredictable and are often caused by unexpected mode changes and system failures. Ground simulation is the only place where it is safe to introduce a pilot to many conditions that may produce these events. Because of this restriction, eventually a high fidelity mock-up with actual hardware should be coupled with the pilot-in-the-loop aircraft ground simulation. This mock-up should include significant pilot cues (e.g., vision system, inceptors, and displays). Structured testing, as already described, can then be used to minimize the risk of adverse APC characteristics lurking in the system design.

Guided by the structured analysis matrix for system performance discussed earlier, maneuvers to evaluate handling qualities throughout all portions of the flight envelope should include the following:

- takeoffs
- landings and go-arounds in various atmospheric conditions (including carrier, short runway, or slope landings, when appropriate)
- aborted takeoffs and landings
- trims and speed offsets
- stalls and pushovers
- wind up turns (i.e., turns conducted with a constant "g" while allowing airspeed to fall off until the aircraft stalls or encounters some other limiting condition)
- configuration changes (flaps, speedbrakes, gear, and thrust) during normal and, in selected cases, off-normal flight conditions
- open-loop inputs (controller pulses and steps, frequency sweeps)
- turn entries
- sideslips
- engine-out conditions
- maneuvering into and out of buffet at high altitude

- mission-oriented precision tasks (e.g., air-to-air tracking, air-to-air refueling, etc.)
- evasive maneuvering

The design and development process is iterative in nature. Design goals may be refined in the course of control law development and analysis and by design changes in response to data updates (e.g., aerodynamics, propulsion, and structures) or other design changes.

Flying qualities evaluations involving piloted simulations are used to validate the FCS design and optimize predicted flying qualities prior to flight testing. Flight test evaluations provide, of course, the final measure of performance. In reality, both simulator and flight-test pilot evaluations can and do lead to design changes. Consideration should be given to the use of both ground-based and in-flight simulator evaluations. In-flight simulator evaluations can be valuable when new functions or fundamental changes in control strategies are planned.

Tasks to Identify APC Tendencies

As a first principle, all evaluation and assessment processes, whether conducted in analysis, simulation, or flight stages, should be designed to actively seek latent APC conditions. Pilot evaluations for APC tendencies should increase the pilot gain or workload and so increase the possibility of finding hidden APC tendencies. Table 4-2 is a composite list of tasks designed to create a sense of extreme urgency and result in high pilot-vehicle gain and aggressive control techniques. For some of these tasks, performance objectives are indicated when a reasonable rationale is available. For military aircraft, the proposed revisions to MIL-STD-1797[70,71] serve this purpose.

In most cases, task-induced stress can be magnified by adding turbulence and wind shears. In addition, the pilot should be instructed to perform the tasks aggressively and accept little error; assessments should emphasize performance, as well as possible APC tendencies. This type of evaluation is sometimes referred to as "handling qualities during tracking" (HQDT).

Most of the tasks in Table 4-2 apply to detecting Category I or II APC events. Category III and non-oscillatory APC events are very difficult to uncover because they are frequently associated with changes in aircraft characteristics due to failures, external inputs, or unexpected mode transitions. A promising test and evaluation technique currently in development by Saab is comprised of a formal procedure of stick movements that successfully revealed APC susceptibilities associated with a buildup of "disconnects" between the pilot's commands and the response of the control surface. This technique has been referred to as the "klonk method" and is described as follows:[19]

TABLE 4-2 Suggested Tasks and Inputs for APC Evaluation

Aggressive Acquisition Maneuvers

Air-to-air and air-to-ground gross acquisition; the acquisition should be as rapid as possible, with overshoots no greater than 5 mils.

Small, precisely controlled heading changes of a specified value (e.g., 10 degrees) using an exactly specified bank angle.

Rapid pitch attitude acquisition in air.

Rapid pitch attitude acquisition after touchdown.

Lineup on very short final approach after breakout.

Rapid shifts in aim point.

Aggressive Tracking Maneuvers

Air-to-air and air-to-ground fine tracking; keep pipper* within 3 to 5 mils of the target for a specified number of seconds.

Pitch attitude tracking in air (in conjunction with attitude acquisition tasks).

Pitch attitude tracking after touchdown (in conjunction with attitude acquisition tasks).

Constant altitude runway fly-bys (~ 5 feet).

Mode Transitions

Autopilot overrides and disconnects at marginal flight conditions (e.g., during extreme turbulence or wind shears).

Detailed examinations of mode shifts that change effective aircraft dynamics; scenarios should be specific to the FCS being tested, including all mode shifts due to configuration changes, air-ground interfaces, failures, etc.

Formation Flying and Aerial Refueling

Close formation (e.g., excursions no greater than ±2 feet from the formation position).

Probe-and-drogue aerial refueling—hook-up without touching the basket webbing.

Boom tracking aerial refueling—keep the pipper within 5 mils of boom nozzle.

Approach and Landing

Lateral offset approaches and landings, including runway shifts; acquire the glide slope and localizer with no more than a specified overshoot; regulate flight path within ±0.1 degrees after acquisition.

Abused landings, last-instant breakouts, lack of go-around option, crew conflict, and other highly unlikely but highly stressful occurrences that may trigger an APC event and/or pilot overcontrol.

Spot landings, including last instant shifts due to factors such as runway incursions or sudden recognition of debris on the runway.

Spot landings with carrier approach or short-takeoff technique (i.e., no flare and extremely precise control) in the presence of burble, turbulence, etc., induced by the carrier's island and stack.

Special Tracking Tasks with Random Forcing Functions

Longitudinal and lateral attitude tracking tasks with random-appearing forcing functions, such as sums of sinusoids, which can be provided as inputs to cockpit displays or as target motions in the external visual field; this approach, which is intended to provide well defined surrogates for a wide variety of specific tracking tasks, offers important advantages, such as (1) providing an exact knowledge of the system forcing function; (2) permitting a workload-graded series of inputs; and (3) allowing PVS dynamics to be directly measured so that the actual dynamic performance is known.

Tests using Adaptable Target Lighting Array System and Ground Attack Test Equipment, which can provide graded workload levels and direct measures. These tests use tracking tasks, references, etc., that can be mechanized in visual systems, including head-up displays, for either ground or in-flight simulations; they are also suitable as a ground target when pertinent.[29]

Longitudinal and lateral attitude regulation, which is similar to the tracking tasks above except that the forcing functions are introduced as external disturbances simulating extreme turbulence.

1. Move the control stick to maximum positive pitch deflection and hold for a selected time period. This is klonk #1.
2. Move the stick to maximum negative pitch deflection and hold until the aircraft reaches maximum positive pitch angle (as a result of the command from the previous step). This is klonk #2.
3. Move the stick to maximum positive pitch deflection and hold until the aircraft reaches maximum negative pitch angle (as a result of the command from the previous step). This is klonk #3.
4. Repeat steps 2 and 3 for the desired number of klonks. For example a 10-klonk test would cycle the pitch stick into the stops a total of 10 times.
5. Simultaneously with steps 1 through 4, move the stick to the maximum left roll position each time the stick is moved to maximum pitch position, and move the stick to the maximum right roll position each time the stick is moved to the minimum pitch position. Also, while the stick is being held in the pitch stops in steps 1 through 4, slowly reduce the roll command at a constant, selected rate.
6. Determine if the aircraft has remained stable and controllable for the specified number of klonks.
7. Repeat steps 1 through 6 using different values for the initial hold period in step 1 and the roll command rate in step 5.

The klonk method has been effective for assessing the effects of the kinds of delay buildup described in Chapter 2 in connection with the second JAS 39 accident.

Flight Test

Many of the tasks for simulator use should be repeated during flight tests. If unexpected APC events are encountered in flight tests, they should be reevaluated in the simulator. It is essential that a significant number of pilots be exposed to the system, during both simulation and flight test evaluations, to ensure that the aircraft will accommodate a wide range of piloting skills. Particular attention should be paid to each pilot's comments during the first exposure to the aircraft. Test pilots, in particular, adapt very quickly and unconsciously to compensate for possible FCS deficiencies.

The selection of pilots for flight (and simulator) testing can be a key factor in developing an APC-free aircraft. Boeing's experience with the 777 indicates that exposure of the aircraft to a large number of pilots can be fruitful in ferreting out problems. In several instances, the first encounter with a particular variety of PIO was discovered with customer, rather than company, test pilots. Once an APC susceptibility was discovered, company test pilots were usually able to duplicate the events, thereby helping to isolate causes and evaluate corrective measures. Airbus, which has by far the largest number of FBW-equipped commercial aircraft in service (more than 600 aircraft, with more than six million flight hours as of early 1996), also emphasizes the need for a diverse pilot population for APC evaluations. For APC clearance, Airbus attempts to include evaluations by three kinds of pilots: (1) pilots who are unfamiliar with the aircraft; (2) test pilots who are "not APC prone" (and, as a result, have little or no experience with APC events, even when flying aircraft with poor APC characteristics); and (3) pilots who are experienced with APCs and can translate their experimental assessments into terms that line pilots can appreciate.

APC-free aircraft require specific examinations and searches for APC tendencies very early in programs, especially in simulations and even in some flight testing operations. These "discovery" processes are aided enormously if at least one pilot has a "high gain" piloting style and an "explorer" attitude and is permitted to engage in carefree flight operations that emphasize the types of tasks and inputs suggested in Table 4-2. As exemplified by the Navy tests for the F-14 backup flight control module described in Chapter 2, the pathway to a flying qualities cliff may not be found using incremental advances from one stabilized flight condition to another. Needless to say, such operations and freedom are seldom popular with program managers. But when they are conducted prudently they can be highly productive.

A general caveat may be appropriate at this point. Hands-on exposure to adverse APC events in training is highly desirable for flight test pilots and engineers. Committee members who were so exposed using an in-flight simulator (see Chapter 5) underscore the need for APC awareness training and for effective learning tools. (It may also be possible to use ground-based simulators for APC awareness training, especially for Category I APC events, but they are not likely to make the same sort of dramatic impression on pilots as in-flight experiences.) APC awareness training does not currently exist within the FAA, and greater emphasis is needed within the Department of Defense.

TECHNICAL FIXES

Careful implementation of recommended processes does not guarantee that APC problems will never be encountered during subsequent analysis and evaluation tests. When problems are encountered, individual analysis will be needed to determine causes and corrective actions. Technical fixes for some of the more common problems include the following:

- Reduce coupling between flexible modes and pilot inputs. Command filtering (e.g., notch filters) may be used to reduce the sensitivity of the PVS to flexible mode coupling. Command filtering has been used to reduce or eliminate oscillations in the 3-Hz regime for the CH-53E helicopter and the Boeing 777 (see, e.g., Nelson and Landes[54]). An unfortunate side effect of such filtering is an additional time delay between the pilot's input and the aircraft's response. If necessary, techniques such as phase stabilization can be used to reduce time delays.

- Mitigate the effect of actuator rate limits. The maximum rate available from the actuator in a control system is often lower than the designer would prefer. Signals to the actuator that demand a higher rate than is available result in an additional delay between the pilot and the actuator response. This has been a primary factor in several Category II and III PIOs and non-oscillatory APC events. The preferred solution is to ensure, by design, that commands cannot exceed the available rate capability. Other solutions are also available, for example a nonlinear scheme for the JAS-39.[60]
- Eliminate integrator windup. "Integrator windup" describes a condition where an integrator in the command path continues to compute even though the element receiving the integrator signal has reached a position or rate limit. When the command to the integrator is reversed, the integrator must unwind before the downstream element will respond. This is another potential source of significant delays between the pilot and the desired aircraft response. A solution to this is to limit the integrator so that the output is less than the actuator displacement minus the sum of any required augmentation signals.

SUMMARY OF FUTURE CONSIDERATIONS

Developing and implementing more effective processes will be complicated because the nature of the problem will continue to evolve as advanced military technologies migrate into civilian aircraft. In addition to FBW and fly-by-light technology, technologies that could make this migration include multiuse control surface effectors (see Chapter 2); all-electric actuation systems; and increasingly complex, unconventional flight control laws, such as "task-tailored" control laws that are optimized for specific flight conditions and tasks.

In addition, commercial aircraft manufacturers have been developing and introducing new technologies and features that have not been used in military aircraft. The commercial use of these technologies has the potential to introduce unique phenomena for which proven APC criteria and analysis methods may not be available. As the number of commercial aircraft that employ these technologies increases, their potential impact also increases. Critical items of interest include the following:

- *Automated modes and pilot proficiency*. As discussed in Chapter 2, current and future airline operations have relied and will continue to rely heavily on automated modes of the FCS. This can lead to very little hand-flying by the pilot, thereby reducing pilot proficiency in manual flying. Adopting unconventional manual flight handling characteristics, which have been proposed for some future aircraft, would further exacerbate APC problems because it would increase the challenge faced by pilots who must quickly assume manual control of the aircraft.
- *Novel inceptor characteristics*. Small-displacement, low-force inceptors are already used on some military and commercial aircraft. They may become more prevalent on future commercial airliners as cockpit designers strive to reduce the weight, size, and volume of control inceptors. Differences have also appeared in the degree to which automatic system operations, such as autothrottles, are reflected in inceptor motions. However, as noted earlier in this chapter, these inceptor characteristics can significantly affect the design process, methods of evaluation, and situation awareness. Without adequate criteria or data, flying qualities designers will not have adequate information to ensure that the characteristics of new inceptors will not contribute to adverse APC.
- *Structural modes*. Reducing the weight of structures reduces the overall weight of the aircraft and improves fuel economy, which are important design goals. However, as optimized structures become more flexible, the structural mode frequencies are reduced, and the potential for an APC event is significantly increased. This trend has already become important in large helicopters and at least one large transport. The APC problems experienced in these aircraft have been countered thus far by notch or low-pass filtering in the command pathway. Limitations in this approach will be reached when the additional time lag associated with this filtering is reflected in poorer flying qualities.
- *Inexperienced designers*. Current trends in the aviation industry will result in fewer and fewer new aircraft developments, which will make it difficult to maintain a cadre of designers with extensive experience in a variety of aircraft and aircraft types. This situation emphasizes the need for specialized training to acquaint designers with APC phenomena (because they will have fewer opportunities to pick up such knowledge in the normal course of events).
- *Software and hardware updates*. Mild APC events can often occur when a pilot is learning the characteristics of a new aircraft. More severe events can occur if there are sudden changes in effective aircraft dynamics. The possibilities of both of these occurrences can

increase significantly if software and hardware updates are not managed properly.

- *Software updates*. Modifications to digital FCSs that include radical control law changes can be implemented by software updates, and the potential for introducing adverse APC characteristics will continue to grow as more and more commercial aircraft are equipped with digital FCSs. Manufacturers and regulatory authorities should redouble current efforts to ensure that (1) software updates are adequately tested, (2) new control laws are compatible with pilots' experience and expectations, and (3) pilots receive necessary training before they are assigned to aircraft with updated software. New, more efficient, more affordable processes could help achieve these goals.
- *Hardware updates*. Aircraft operating lifetimes are now generally far longer than the technological lifetime of digital FCS equipment. Major investments are made in software validation and verification, some of which are hardware specific. Significant incompatibilities and significant additional costs can be anticipated in the future as FCSs are replaced and associated software is reworked.

5

Simulation and Analysis of the Pilot-Vehicle System

The most important design tools for avoiding, discovering, understanding, and correcting APC events are simulation and analysis. Although the emphasis is on avoidance, discovery (or lack thereof) is the central issue. To avoid or discover APC problems, a competent design team must be guided by past experience and the effective use of simulation and analysis tools.

Because attaining experience on one's own can be very expensive, experiences of others—revealed in lore, criteria, research reports, and papers—can be invaluable. Simulation and analysis, which work most efficiently as complementary enterprises, usually operate at different levels and with different priorities either during the development of an aircraft or in solving APC problems that unexpectedly appear in flight. Thus, analysis early in the development process is central to the following enterprises: delineating which potential effective aircraft dynamics are prone to adverse APC; providing a window for discovering or forecasting potential problem areas; and determining areas and issues to be addressed by piloted simulations.

Analysis includes computer simulations without actual pilots, although they may be represented by pilot models. In full-scale development, however, piloted simulation is the primary tool for understanding and correcting flight-discovered APC events. Pilot-vehicle analysis continues to be an important aid as development continues.

By its very nature, piloted simulation deals in specific situations, whereas pilot-vehicle analysis can provide a basis for extrapolation and interpolation. At any stage of aircraft development, judicious pilot-vehicle analysis can be of immense help in reducing the number of vehicle configurations that should be evaluated to declare an aircraft design free of APC tendencies. Joint simulation and PVS analysis may be used to select configurations and piloting tasks that appear to be prone to APC problems. A subset of configurations can then be subjected to further simulation and possible flight tests to reduce the risk of undiscovered APC tendencies.

The state of the art in both piloted simulation and pilot-vehicle analysis is rapidly advancing, so what might have been doctrine yesterday may be outdated today. At present, the interpretation of piloted simulation, aided and guided by analysis, is the major factor in the design and assessment of APC-free PVSs. Nevertheless, simulation and analysis are not yet suitable for the unambiguous clearance of an aircraft as APC-free. That can only be demonstrated in flight. Indeed, experience has shown that only after many flights with many pilots that have included all possible maneuvers in the presence of all possible flight environments can one speak with assurance of an APC-free aircraft. Thus, it seems that a residual probability of experiencing an APC event continues throughout the life of an aircraft fleet.

In the following sections, the use of piloted simulations is discussed in more detail. This is followed by a discussion of PVS modeling features that are especially relevant to reducing the risk of APC events.

GROUND AND IN-FLIGHT SIMULATION

A number of simulation tools are available during the development of an aircraft. These tools can be ranked in terms of their "fidelity" to actual in-flight conditions. Fidelity in piloted simulation is defined as "the degree to which characteristics of perceivable states induce realistic pilot psychomotor and cognitive behavior for a given task and environment."[2] Fidelity in this sense relates primarily to the effect upon the pilot—not to the effective aircraft dynamics—although both aspects are necessarily involved. The simulation tools usually available during development are described below.

Non-Real-Time Simulators. The pilots in the loop are represented by pilot models. Thus, these simulators typically have low fidelity for pilot behavior. However, the fidelity can be very high for the effective aircraft dynamics, including flexible modes, etc.

Ground-Based, Pilot-in-the-Loop, Fixed-Base and Moving-Base Simulators. Typically, fixed-base and moving-base simulators for a specific aircraft can accurately reproduce the cockpit station (including displays and inceptors) and the extended rigid-body effective aircraft characteristics. Motion cues are either nonexistent (fixed-base) or are contaminated by washout filters* and other motion-limiting elements (moving-base). Visual cues can be excellent for up-and-away flight but may still not reproduce the high resolution and texture required for low-altitude flying.

In-Flight Simulators. Unless an in-flight simulator is specifically designed for a particular cockpit and inceptors, the pilot-related fidelity may be limited. However, the extended rigid-body effective vehicle dynamics may be well approximated, and motion and visual cues may be superior to the best ground-based simulators.

"Hot-Bench" and "Iron-Bird" Simulators. These two kinds of simulators, which are described below, offer high fidelity to actual flight hardware. They can be coupled to ground-based, pilot-in-the-loop simulations for a broad range of explorations.

Prototype and Developmental Test Aircraft. These aircraft offer true fidelity if they are full scale. The quality of assessments of flying qualities decreases as the amount of scaling increases. Prototypes and test aircraft also have extensive data sensing and recording capabilities thereby providing an excellent basis for studying APC possibilities. However, their high cost and importance to the program may militate against the aggressive pursuit of hazardous APC phenomena. Also, the number of pilots is often limited.

Operational Vehicles. These vehicles have true fidelity and are operated by a large pilot population, but they have limited data recording capability.

The tools described above can be ranked according to overall fidelity, depending on the nature of the specific tasks involved. Invariably, non-real-time simulations are considered to have the lowest fidelity, while prototype, development, and operational vehicles are considered to have the highest. The availability of these tools also differs greatly, with lower fidelity tools being more available than higher fidelity tools.

Despite the high incentive and cost benefits of uncovering potential APC problems as early as possible, significant APC problems are often not discovered until flight testing a prototype or operational aircraft, during which solutions can be both expensive and time consuming. Ideally, APC problems can be eliminated by design at the very beginning or, at least, discovered in mid-design phases that primarily depend on ground-based simulations. It is crucial to determine the tasks and level of fidelity necessary to maximize the effectiveness of ground-based simulations.

SIMULATION TYPES

Non-Real-Time Simulations

An off-line, non-real time simulation model is usually employed first in any aircraft development program. This simulation model can be developed and used at an office or laboratory computer work station and involves none of the "virtual reality" requirements of a simulation with an actual pilot in the loop. The model of the effective vehicle dynamics can be quite complex and can include many system nonlinearities attributable to either vehicle aerodynamics or control system implementations. This kind of off-line simulation is often used to develop mathematical models for pilot-in-the-loop simulations.

Non-real-time simulations can be used in a variety of ways to support an APC analysis. Because the simulations can have fairly accurate representations of the control system actuators and nonlinearities, such as FCS rate and position limiting, non-real-time simulations can explore the likelihood and extent of non-oscillatory APC events with inputs from cockpit control inceptors. The potential for all categories of PIOs can also be examined with the aid of simple, pure-gain, pilot models (see the Synchronous Pilot Model section, below). In addition, a number of other relatively simple techniques for uncovering PIO-prone aircraft and flight conditions have also been proposed.[65] These off-line, non-real-time simulations can be exceptionally valuable for mapping areas and parameters of concern and for planning more elaborate simulations with real pilots.

Pilot-in-the-Loop, Fixed-Base Simulation

The question of whether or not pilot-in-the-loop, fixed-base simulation with no simulated motion cues can reliably uncover APC tendencies is still being fervently debated. In fact, several committee members expressed fiercely held opinions on this subject. The consensus that evolved is outlined below.

Some researchers and practitioners believe that motion cues are not important in ground-based simulators because they never actually duplicate the motion cues of the real aircraft and because pilots learn to filter out or ignore motion cues in flight. (In fact, the latter is an important attribute of successful instrument flight). Proponents of this point of view believe realistic visual cues free from noticeable time delays are of greater value. As an example, the excellent visual cues provided in large-screen (i.e., IMAX®) theaters provide outstanding motion sensation with no actual motion.

NASA used fixed-base simulators to investigate the Shuttle Orbiter PIO incident that occurred in an early flight test of an unpowered, full-scale prototype[20] (see Table 1-2). NASA concluded that by carefully tailoring the tracking tasks in the fixed-base simulator it could be used to evaluate candidate control-system modifications. But this was possible only after the PIO had occurred in flight. In other words, pre-flight simulation had not been useful for predicting APC susceptibility. Although the state of the art has advanced since then, the situation has not changed much in this regard.

In the investigations of the famous T-38 PIO recorded in Figure 1-1, fixed-base simulations were also useful for making some qualitative evaluations but were not successful in duplicating the PIO.[35] This is not surprising, because the bobweight effect, which depends upon cockpit motion for its existence, was ultimately demonstrated to be an important factor. It is noteworthy that the Lockheed Martin YF-22 incident described in Chapter 2 could *not* be reproduced in a fixed-base simulator, despite the fact that numerous pilots flew the accident profile and that the precise conditions surrounding this incident were known.[11]

Based on these and similar experiences, many experts question using fixed-base simulation to discover and eliminate adverse APC tendencies. Many reasons have been put forth to justify this position, including the absence of flight-induced stress, time lags in the visual display system, the lack of effective visual and motion cues, simulation artifacts, and poor fidelity to the actual aircraft. This committee, however, is convinced that properly configured fixed-base simulations can be reliable indicators of many potential adverse APC tendencies. This viewpoint is shared by many designers and investigators who use state-of-the-art fixed-base simulations that faithfully replicate aircraft performance. For instance, Gibson[23] comments upon the fixed-base simulation techniques used for many years by British Aerospace at Warton:

> The oscillation from the FBW Jaguar digital FCS research aircraft shows how powerful is the attraction to the "PIO frequency" (nominally where the attitude lags the stick by 180 degrees) even for the most minute amplitudes. Extreme variations in attitude close to the ground would be stupefying. A subtle control strategy could not be expected. It is also unnecessary to invoke the control of normal acceleration in landing or take-off pitch PIO, and meaningless in roll PIO, which is of generally identical character. Examination of PIO records shows the dominant role of the zero crossings of the attitude rate, representing the peaks in attitude. This point signals the reversal of the stick motion. *Simply by exciting the PIO frequency oscillation at all stick amplitudes including the largest possible, without regard for any task "trigger," it is possible to determine the susceptibility to PIO*. The nature of the stick force and displacement characteristics (which must of course be accurately simulated) tends to induce the variations in shape and phasing [i.e., near sinusoids to more rectangular waveforms]. A conventional pitch stick will tend to produce a sinusoidal input with its peaks locked to the attitude peaks. Shorter travel and/or light forces will tend to produce a more relay-like action, but probably retaining some elements of the sinusoid. A very short travel stick is likely to produce an almost pure relay-like

action with its fundamental apparently locked to the rate peaks.[23] (emphasis added)

Gibson also describes an example in which an aircraft had PIOs in pitch, roll, or both in each of its first five flights.[25] On the sixth flight, a divergent pitch PIO occurred in what was initially a routine landing. The adverse APC that was so blatantly obvious in flight had been found in simulation beforehand but had been dismissed because "pilots wouldn't fly like that." This phrase is heard frequently when unusual APC events appear in simulation and even more often when an analyst finds some peculiar possibilities in pilot-vehicle analysis. "Discoveries" of APC tendencies are seldom popular with schedule-driven engineering managers.

In the Boeing 777 case study (see Chapter 2), the PIO encountered in flight was manifested to the pilot in the simulator in terms of higher workload and reduced task performance and not as a PIO. Higher workload and reduced performance features, often coupled with the pilot's sense that the aircraft's response is not sufficiently predictable, are harbingers of possible APC problems.

In another example, the U.S. Army *Handling Qualities Requirements for Military Rotorcraft* (ADS-33D) has a battery of flight-test evaluation maneuvers that precisely define standards for precision and levels of aggressiveness.[68] These standards were used extensively during evaluations of the LHX helicopter and did, in fact, predict APC problems that were later confirmed in a flight test vehicle. In fact, it is interesting to note that the flight test vehicle had been flown by many pilots without observing adverse APC tendencies. Only after flights were performed according to the ADS-33D specification to validate the simulator results were APC events actually observed in flight.

Many of the committee members and technical liaisons to the committee have been intimately involved with developing aircraft FCSs, including piloted simulations, and their combined experience covers dozens of aircraft. These individuals are aware of many cases in which simulations exhibited characteristics that, if left uncorrected, could have led to APC events. In these cases, the fixed-base simulation exercises did just what they were intended to do. A great many potential problems were corrected during the development process and became non-events in flight testing.

The committee is also aware of situations in which unsatisfactory simulation results did not result in corrective action (often because the unsatisfactory results were associated with tasks that were viewed as uncharacteristic of actual flight operations). In many of these cases, the problem subsequently resurfaced as a full-fledged APC event. Thus, although in some cases APCs are not predicted by piloted simulations, in other cases, they occurred when signs of potential trouble were ignored. Finally, for whatever reasons, the potential for APC events sometimes escapes detection in the simulation process, which often results in APC events, such as the YF-22 accident, that have a high degree of visibility. The exaggerated criticism—that the simulation process is not effective—rather than less than 100 percent effective—is unfortunate because it tends to impugn the overall efficacy of simulation.

This discussion has focused attention on four essential features of fixed-based simulation that are required for it to be an effective tool for identifying adverse APC tendencies:

- Tasks must be identified that are difficult enough to stress the PVS, even if these tasks are not necessarily "realistic."
- There must be recognition that a PVS oscillation is not the only indicator of a potential APC problem. Other indicators include substantially increased workload, reduced performance, and lack of predictability of responses.
- Pilot ratings indicating degradation among effective vehicle dynamics are more gradual and less distinct in the fixed-base environment than in moving-base or in-flight simulations.
- The fixed-base simulation, including inceptors, visual scene, and display characteristics, should be as close to the controlled element dynamics and effective aircraft dynamics as possible, and the differences should be quantified. For example, pitch-attitude/pilot-inceptor transfer characteristics should be measured and compared with the properties expected in the actual aircraft.

Pilot-in-the-Loop, Moving-Base and In-Flight Simulation

Historical Perspectives. Because moving-base simulators have the capability of emulating motion, at least to a limited extent, they would appear to be more powerful tools for assessing APC susceptibility than fixed-base simulators. However, the utility of these devices has also been called into question. Figure 5-1 compares a group of four simulators used in NASA's investigation of the Shuttle PIO incident alluded to earlier.[59] The Flight Simulator for Advanced Aircraft was a moving-base simulator (no longer in existence) capable of large lateral translations. The Vertical Motion Simulator is capable of large vertical translations. The Total In-Flight Simulator is a highly modified C-131 transport. In the Shuttle APC investigation, PIO susceptibility ratings (using the PIO rating scale shown in Figure 5-2) were obtained on the moving-base and in-flight simulators for various tasks (see Figures 5-3, 5-4, and 5-5). With its ability to provide high fidelity visual and motion cues, the Total In-Flight Simulator provided PIO ratings that more closely reflected those of the actual Shuttle vehicle in normal landings, with and without lateral offsets. By artificially increasing the task difficulty, the moving-base simulators exhibited some improvement in predicting APCs.

A general conclusion about these simulators is that, once an APC tendency has been observed in flight, it is possible to construct a piloting task that will exhibit the same tendencies in ground-based simulation. In addition, as simulator fidelity increases (e.g., moving versus fixed-base, in-flight versus ground-based), APC tendencies noted in flight can be reproduced with piloting tasks that are more realistic. Finally, and perhaps most importantly, as simulated piloting tasks become more realistic, simulation results are more likely to influence the program personnel responsible for allocating resources to investigate and alleviate potential APC problems.

Recent Experience. Several committee members and technical liaisons visited the Calspan Corporation in Buffalo, New York, to discuss APC phenomena and participate in APC demonstrations in a modified Learjet test aircraft with variable stability. A valuable demonstration was given of how the characteristics of an APC-prone aircraft could go undetected during normal operations and then dramatically surface when a high-gain task was attempted by the pilot. This experience is described below.

	Simulator			
Capability	Fixed-Base	FSAA	VMS	TIFS
Aerodynamic Model	6 DOF Nonlinear	6 DOF Nonlinear	6 DOF Nonlinear	6 DOF Nonlinear
Visual Display	Limited	TV model-board	TV model-board	"Actual"
Motion	None	Good for small amplitude	Good for small and large amplitude	Complete
Principal Piloting Task(s)	Tracking (tailored)	1. Landing 2. Tracking	Large disturbance landings	Full set

FIGURE 5-1 A comparison of NASA and U.S. Air Force simulators for principal piloting tasks, circa 1975. Source: Powers.[59]

DOF = degree of freedom
FSAA = Flight Simulator for Advanced Aircraft
TIFS = Total In-Flight Simulator
VMS = Vertical Motion Simulator

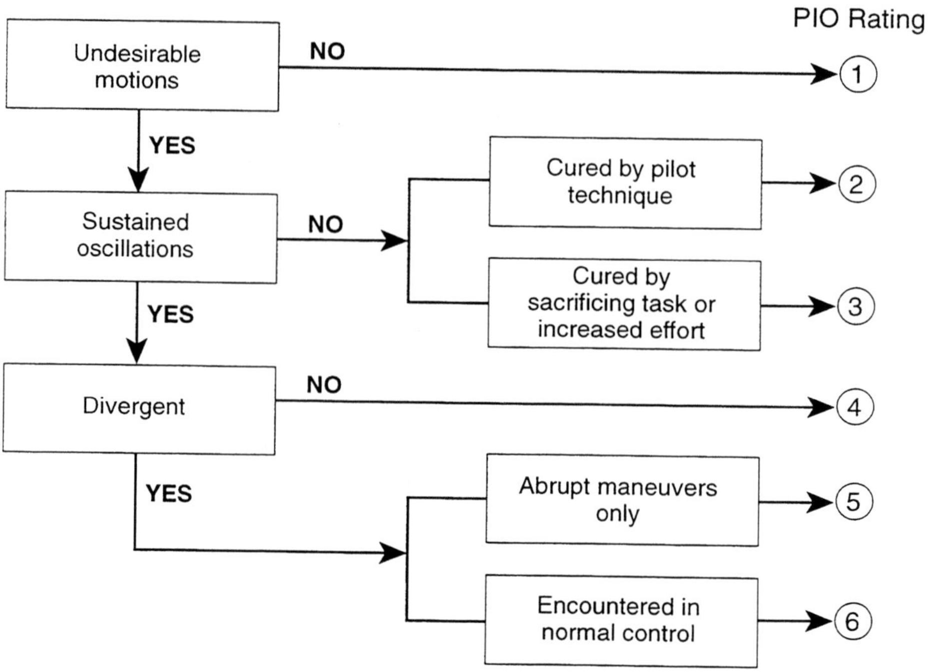

FIGURE 5-2 A PIO (APC) rating scale. Source: Powers.[59]

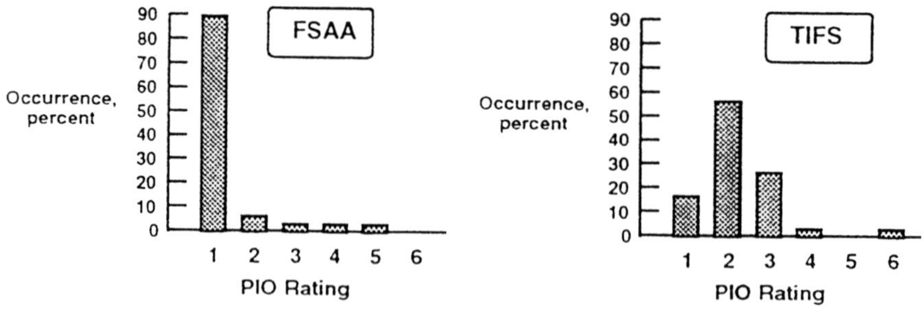

FIGURE 5-3 A comparison of PIO ratings showing normal and offset landing tasks by the NASA Flight Simulator for Advanced Aircraft (FSAA) and the U.S. Air Force Total In-Flight Simulator (TIFS). Source: Powers.[59]

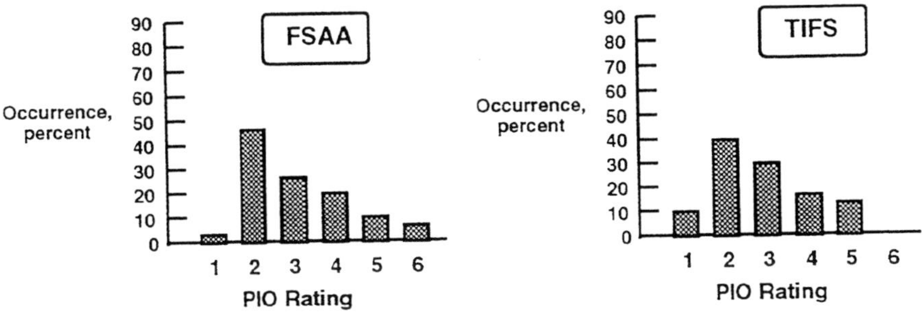

FIGURE 5-4 A comparison of PIO ratings for formation-flying by the NASA Flight Simulator for Advanced Aircraft (FSAA) and the U.S. Air Force Total In-Flight Simulator (TIFS). Source: Powers.[59]

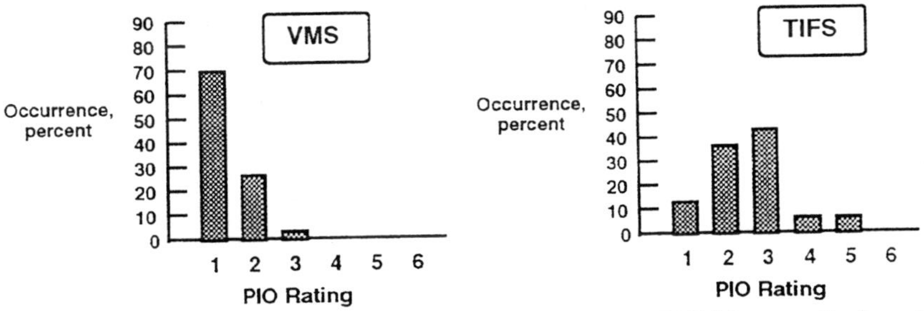

*** 150-ft lateral offset at 100-ft above runway, and 15-ft/sec vertical gust at 50-ft above runway**

Figure 5-5 A comparison of PIO ratings for demanding landing tasks by the NASA vertical motion simulator (VMS) and the U.S. Air Force total in-flight simulator (TIFS). Source: Powers, 1984.[59]

A number of approaches were flown to the Niagara Falls airport in which the pilot initially aligned the aircraft to land in a ditch parallel to, but 300 feet offset from, the runway. During the approach, at an altitude of about 150 feet above the runway, the instructor pilot called for the flying pilot to maneuver the aircraft to land on the runway within a predetermined normal touchdown zone. This required aggressive manipulation of the controls, but the task was easily accomplished as long as the aircraft FCS was in its normal configuration.

When the FCS was modified to simulate less-responsive surface actuators, the aircraft flew in a normal manner until the high-gain task was called for. At that point, the aggressive action of the pilot rate-saturated the FCS, which resulted in an APC very close to the ground. The APC was terminated by the instructor pilot executing a missed approach. This change in aircraft behavior was described by the instructor pilot as a flying-qualities cliff. On a subsequent approach with the same FCS configuration, the pilot modified his actions to avoid the flying qualities cliff, demonstrating the possibility of avoiding an APC problem once the potential for the problem is known.

Demonstrations like this are necessary to train test pilots to determine the APC potential of aircraft and to inform line pilots that APC events may be associated with FCS deficiencies rather than with poor piloting. It is extremely important that line pilots understand that flight characteristics of APC-prone aircraft can change and that they must modify their gains to accommodate the FCS. Pilots should understand that different pilots can have different gains at different times, and it may be possible for one pilot to control an aircraft in circumstances that could lead to an accident with another pilot.

If an aircraft has an APC tendency, sooner or later someone will encounter a problem. Pilots naturally hesitate to admit they have problems flying an aircraft that other pilots have flown without difficulty. With an APC-prone aircraft, the superior test pilot is the one who can detect a problem. A line pilot who discovers an APC characteristic may prevent a tragedy by sharing that information. Thus, it is important to educate both test pilots and line pilots about APCs and to encourage them to report suspected APC events.

Hot-Bench and Iron-Bird Simulation

Hot-bench simulations use actual flight hardware (flight computers, actuators, control surfaces, etc.), rather than simulations that employ mathematical models of these components. If the components just described are located in a frame that replicates their locations on the real aircraft, and if the actuators are subject to simulated aerodynamic loads, the name iron bird is applied to the simulation. Hot-bench and iron-bird simulations are used to verify hardware performance. Their utility in the assessment of a vehicle's susceptibility to APC problems includes verification that the performance requirements and specifications of various flight control subsystems have been met before flight and ensuring that control model switching (e.g., from a primary FBW FCS to a backup mechanical FCS) produces no unwanted transients that could serve as APC triggers. Hot-bench and iron-bird simulations can also be part of pilot-in-the-loop, fixed-base simulation studies that serve as fundamental tools for validating detailed FCS properties, especially in nonlinear regimes. Hot-bench and iron-bird simulations may also be "vehicles" used to develop key describing functions to support some FCS and PVS analyses.

Simulation Summary

The subject of pilot-in-the-loop simulation cannot be left without pointing out the small but finite probability that ground simulators (especially moving-base simulators) might produce APC events attributable to the limitations of the simulator rather than to deficiencies in the aircraft being simulated. These are often referred to as artifacts of the simulation process. Foremost among simulator limitations are the computational time delays that accrue in generating digital scenes and the necessity of using washout filters and attenuating motion amplitude in the system that provides the simulator cab motion.

The deleterious effects of time delays in actual FCSs and their role in APC susceptibility are well known. Indeed, these delays contribute significantly to the frequency-dependent phase lags described in Chapter 2. Motion washout filters remove the low frequency (large amplitude) components of commanded cab motion, and attenuating motion amplitude further reduces the amplitude of cab motion at all frequencies. But the motion cues the simulation pilot receives are obviously distorted, compared to cues received by a pilot flying the actual vehicle. This distortion can modify pilot behavior in the simulator. It should also be noted that questions about simulator fidelity are sometimes used to explain away anomalies in simulator test results, even when the anomalies are, in fact, characteristic of the system being tested.

Piloted simulations, including fixed-base simulations, have a rich but checkered history as predictors of PIO potential. It is generally recognized that CH PRs (Cooper-Harper pilot ratings) and PIO ratings derived from simulator testing tend to be less discriminating than in-flight ratings, although the trends among comparative configurations may be similar. Ongoing attempts to use simulators to duplicate the severe PIOs from flight tests have shown the following:[5]

- Simulator tests duplicated some—but not all—of the PIOs demonstrated in flight. However, in all cases aircraft configurations that demonstrated severe PIO characteristics in flight exhibited PIO tendencies in the simulations for all pilots.
- CH PRs and PIO ratings obtained in the simulators indicated somewhat better aircraft performance than flight tests.
- Simulators indicated major differences in workloads and ease of control between configurations that were demonstrated to be PIO-prone and baseline configurations that were free of PIOs.

In short, simulator test results include many key features necessary to assess PIO potential accurately, but the cues and clues are more subtle and less distinct than they are in flight tests.

OVERVIEW OF HUMAN PILOT CHARACTERISTICS

Modern Piloting Tasks

Modern flight control and navigation systems are characterized by two features: (1) they employ FBW controls, and (2) they introduce extensive automation support into the cockpit, ranging from complex SASs in manual control modes to powerful flight management computers* and autopilots that assume responsibility for most flight control tasks (and which may operate the aircraft in ways that are difficult for pilots to monitor and understand). These modern systems leave the pilot in a supervisory control mode most of the time. Consequently, crew members monitor, supervise, plan, and, in essence, serve as information managers. Although pilots have experience flying their aircraft manually, they are seldom in active, direct control of the aircraft. However, if a failure or unexpected upset occurs, they are required to assume control immediately. To maintain situational awareness, pilots must be vigilant, continually aware of the state and characteristics of aircraft systems and continually anticipating situations that could compromise the safe operation of the aircraft; good pilots must "keep ahead of their aircraft."

Human Pilot Performance

Pilot performance can be thought of in terms of three steps: perception, decision making, and action. The pilot's *perception* involves sensing and interpreting available information. *Decision making* means the pilot determines what to do next and what control strategy to adopt on the basis of perceptions. Finally, the pilot takes *action* consistent with the perceived or expected world. Modeling human pilot performance has been a goal of engineers and psychologists for more than half a century. This effort has been most successful in modeling pilot performance in continuous flight-control activity. This is precisely the type of activity associated with PIOs, but not necessarily with non-oscillatory APC events.

Pilot action requires that the pilot act as an element in a feedback control system. Figure 5-6 is a stylized representation of this feedback structure, referred to here and elsewhere as the PVS (pilot-vehicle system). In Figure 5-6, the pilot is shown moving a cockpit control stick or inceptor in response to a visually perceived deviation in aircraft pitch attitude from some desired value. The motion of the cockpit inceptor is an input to the flight control computer. On the basis of information about vehicle motion, the computer then determines an appropriate command to apply to the actuator that drives the appropriate control surface, in this case, the elevator. Figure 5-6 is referred to as a feedback system because, when the pilot visually senses aircraft pitch-attitude deviations and responds accordingly, he effectively closes a feedback control loop.

The flight control computer may receive signals from vehicle motion as well as commands generated by the pilot. For example, the flight control computer may form part of a SAS, which eases the pilot's burden or workload in piloting the aircraft. As discussed in Chapter 1 (see Figure 1-2), the combination of SAS and aircraft defines the effective aircraft dynamics, and the characteristics of the effective aircraft help determine susceptibility to APC events.

Although visually sensed aircraft motion is probably the most important feedback mechanism for the pilot from the standpoint of aircraft control, a variety of other feedback variables or cues can be sensed by the pilot. These include motion or vestibular cues that provide information about angular, normal, and lateral velocities and accelerations and proprioceptive cues that provide information about the position of the pilot's own limbs when moving the cockpit inceptor. The human sensors that provide both vestibular and proprioceptive cues inherent in human physiology will not be discussed in detail here. Their effects, however, are implicitly included in pilot models for aircraft control.

Discussions of modeling human behavior invariably give rise to questions concerning human variability, adaptability, and choice. Some of the factors that contribute to pilot variability on a global scale may have a cultural basis. For example, pilots from one culture might tend to quickly disconnect an automated system (such as the autopilot or autothrottle) if they do not understand what it is doing, whereas pilots of another might persist in the belief that automated controls outperform manual control.

The pilot-modeling efforts of direct interest to PIO applications are focused upon very well defined piloting tasks in which human behavior is, by necessity, highly constrained. For example, a well trained, well motivated pilot

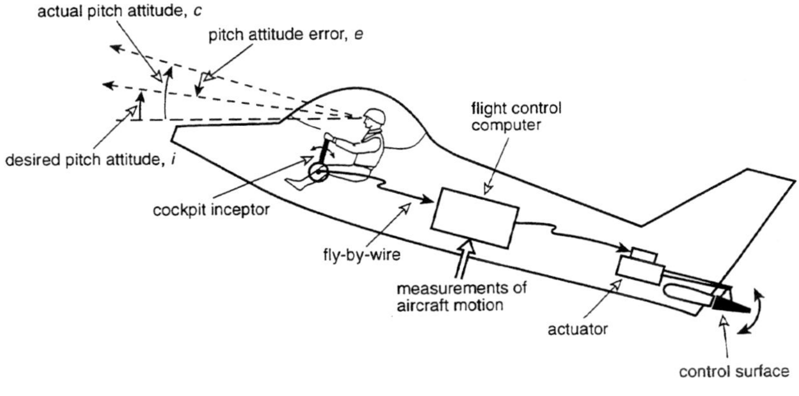

FIGURE 5-6 A feedback system involving the human pilot.

engaged in landing a large commercial aircraft is constrained by the task and environment to the extent that the pilot's behavior and performance can often be adequately described by what is referred to as a "describing function model."[34,44] In its complete incarnation, such a model describes both the pilot's "linear behavior" (i.e., behavior that could be replicated by a relatively simple inanimate control device with linear characteristics), and the pilot's "nonlinear behavior" (i.e., behavior that can be attributed to the complex, nonlinear sensing and actuation capabilities of a human being).

PILOT MODELS AND PILOT-VEHICLE ANALYSES

Mathematical models of human pilots have been developed along the lines of control theory. Indeed, the control theory paradigm has become the primary way engineers view the human pilot in well defined piloting tasks. It is not surprising, then, that synthesizing models of the human pilot closely parallels synthesizing inanimate controllers in feedback control systems. Just as control-system design techniques can be conveniently partitioned into classical and modern approaches, so can techniques for modeling the pilot. In addition to the classical-modern dichotomy, one can also distinguish pilot models on the basis of their ability to model the physiological subsystems responsible for sensing and actuation (e.g., the sensors of the inner ear that provide human beings with information about self-motion and the neuromuscular combinations that allow precise movement of the limbs).

Classical Approach

Background

Classical control-system design techniques employ frequency-domain synthesis. In simple terms, these techniques transform the variable that describes duration (i.e., time) into one that describes the rapidity of change (i.e., frequency). Because time is such a natural measure, this transformation would seem to obscure the problem. However, the advantages of the frequency domain approach have been known to control system engineers since the 1940s.[6]

In the classical approach, the human pilot is represented by what is referred to as a describing or transfer function.[34,44] The transfer function is a frequency-domain representation that can predict a system's output (in the time or frequency domain) as a function of its input. Figure 5-7 is a block diagram of this cause-effect representation. (This kind of representation was also used in Figure 1-2 in a much more detailed form.) The lines with arrows represent physical, time-varying signals. The directions of the arrows represent cause and effect; the line directed toward the block represents a "cause," or input, and the line directed away from the block represents an "effect," or output. The block itself represents the transfer function of the system in question (e.g., the human pilot).

As an example, referring to Figure 5-6, the input to the pilot could be the time-varying signal that is the difference between the desired and actual aircraft pitch attitude; the output from the pilot could be the time-varying signal that is the cockpit inceptor motion. The use of the word "signal" for the variable in question can be traced to classical control-system design, which began with the work of electrical engineers.[6]

Crossover Model

One of the simplest, but perhaps most profound, models of the human pilot is called the "crossover model." The name derives from the particular frequency range (i.e., the crossover region) in the frequency response diagram of the transfer function for the combined system of the pilot and the controlled element where the model is most accurate. The crossover model effectively describes how a human pilot can adapt to the response characteristics of various aircraft. This model is an archetype of appropriate feedback control operations in that it follows the most fundamental rule of thumb for synthesizing inanimate control systems: the characteristics of the control system are adjusted so that the cause-effect relationship between system error and system output approximates integration in the time domain.

Consider Figure 5-8, where a second block has been added to the diagram in Figure 5-7. The second block represents the characteristics of the aircraft. The crossover model states that the transfer function obtained by a combination (multiplication) of the transfer functions of the pilot and the vehicle in Figure 5-8 will have a very simple form in a limited but important frequency range (called the crossover region). This form, which describes time integration (with a time delay) of the visually-sensed input error, is equivalent to a dynamic system element that includes a time delay (including human reaction time) and produces an output that is the time integral of the delayed input. This model has been applied several times elsewhere in this report.

A number of pilot model formulations can be traced to the crossover model. Some of these reflect feedback associated with detailed neuromuscular physiology. No descriptions of these models will be attempted here. Specific examples of relevant models for high-frequency PIOs can be found in other studies.[33,37]

Synchronous Pilot Model

An examination of the time histories associated with many PIOs indicates that, during a PIO, the cockpit inceptor motion is nearly in phase with, or synchronous with, the vehicle oscillation. This suggests that, in analyzing the PIO, the pilot model can be reduced to a simple gain, with a magnitude that produces incipient instability from the standpoint of control system design. The quotation from Gibson given earlier reflects this form of pilot behavior. In another recent study,[42] the utility of this approach was shown using data from a well documented series of flight tests.[5] The obvious advantage of this approach is that it dramatically simplifies the pilot modeling procedure while simultaneously focusing attention upon the shortcomings of the dynamics of the effective vehicle, which are the underlying causes of the APC. The synchronous pilot model is, without doubt, the most valuable pilot model for providing insight and understanding of fully-developed PIOs. It is also by far the simplest. The synchronous model is also applied elsewhere in this report.

Modern Approach

Background

The advent of powerful computer algorithms to design control systems has led to the development of algorithmic pilot models, which are generated by sophisticated computer-aided-design programs for control-system synthesis. Although the modern approach emphasizes system description in the time domain as opposed to the frequency domain, models in this category can be compared with the classical ones by a simple transformation from one domain to the other.

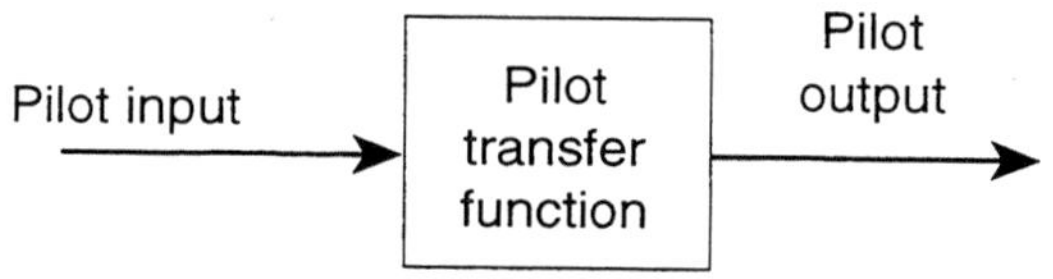

FIGURE 5-7 A block diagram representation of the human pilot transfer function.

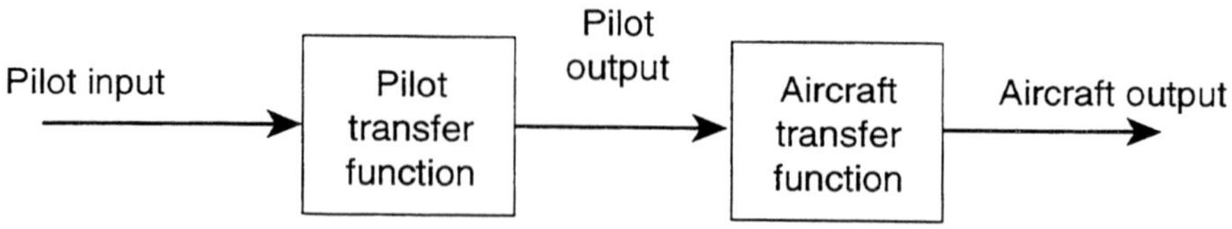

FIGURE 5-8 A block diagram of an open-loop PVS.

Optimal Control Model

One successful example of pilot modeling using the modern approach is the optimal control model (OCM) of the human pilot.[34] The primary hypothesis behind the OCM is that the trained, motivated human pilot behaves in an optimal manner. Thus, in a well defined flight task, the pilot attempts to optimize an inferred performance measure, typically represented by a weighted sum of average control error and average inceptor rate. The latter quantity is often taken as a measure of pilot workload. The optimization of the performance function by means of mathematical algorithms derived from linear optimal control and estimation theory leads to a specific form for the model. (In the parlance of the classical approach, this model would be referred to as a specific transfer function.)

The OCM of the human pilot is well suited to modeling pilot behavior in well controlled experimental conditions, such as those occurring in ground or in-flight simulators. The model is ideally suited to handling multiple pilot cues (e.g., vestibular as well as visual cues) and to modeling pilot activity in which more than one vehicle response is being controlled by the pilot (e.g., controlling aircraft roll attitude as well as pitch attitude). Useful examples of applications of the OCM to pilot modeling can be found in the Handbook of Human Factors and Ergonomics.[34] Unfortunately, because the OCM is based on optimal pilot behavior, it does not reproduce the incipient instability that accompanies APC events. It can, however, be used to estimate pre-transition and long-term post-transition pilot dynamics for Category III PIOs. Pilot rating predictions can also be made from OCM results. Such estimates can show workload changes implicit in the pilot's adaptation to changes in the effective aircraft dynamics. These changes can indicate the difficulties of possible transitions that are candidates for Category III PIO triggers.

Finally, the OCM or a variant can be useful in estimating pilot lead or lag time, which can be used in the Moscow Aviation Institute boundaries (described in Chapter 6).

Different Modes of Pilot Behavior

Compensatory Control

It should be emphasized that, except for the synchronous pilot model, the type of pilot behavior that has been discussed to this point is usually referred to as "compensatory." That is, the pilot senses a discrepancy between a desired state and an actual aircraft state (e.g., pitch attitude), and the pilot compensates for the errors by providing a corrective input. Consider Figure 5-9, which describes a complete feedback system. To explain the diagram in more concrete fashion, assume that the input (i) is a time-varying aircraft pitch-attitude command generated by the flight control computer and displayed electronically to the pilot in the cockpit. The pilot's task is to force the aircraft to follow this command with minimum error. However, in the example, the cockpit display only indicates the system error (e) to the pilot. The situation shown in Figure 5-9 defines the compensatory piloting task in which the pilot's actions respond to system error. Another example of compensatory behavior occurs when a pilot is using the instrument landing system display in the cockpit to conduct a landing. This display provides information regarding aircraft position above or below the desired glide slope.

The exquisite adaptability of the human pilot allows other types of behavior, most of which have been studied and categorized extensively.[44] These are briefly described below.

Pursuit Control

Assume that a display modification in Figure 5-9 is undertaken so that the system input (*i*) and aircraft output (*c*) are displayed in the cockpit, the latter being the actual aircraft pitch attitude. Because both *i* and *c* are now available, the difference (*e*) could also easily be visually extracted by the pilot. If the pilot makes use of this added display information, "pursuit pilot behavior" would be in evidence. The word "pursuit" is used because the pilot's control action can be thought of as being generated by his pursuit of the command signal. That is, the pilot pursues the goal of matching *c* to *i*, thereby minimizing *e*. Under many circumstances, the pilot can actually sense the quantities needed for control and can "develop" his or her own internal pursuit display.

Precognitive Control

There is evidence of another model of pilot behavior that may not involve continuous feedback at all. Once the pilot has become completely familiar with the aircraft response characteristics and the perceptual field, a highly-skilled pilot can, under certain conditions, generate deft, discrete, properly timed, and

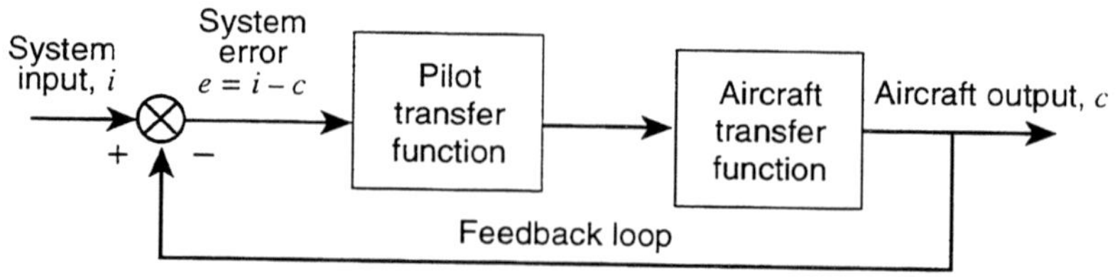

FIGURE 5-9 A block diagram of a closed-loop PVS.

sequenced outputs (i.e., movements of the cockpit inceptor) that result in aircraft responses that are almost exactly the ones desired. This mode of behavior has been referred to as "precognitive" control. Most highly skilled movements that have been thoroughly learned and practiced enough to become automatic (i.e., not requiring conscious thought) fall into this category. Synchronous behavior for sinusoidal inputs is, perhaps, the most common example and is certainly the most important for PIO considerations.

Organization of Perceptions

Given appropriate visual cues, the human pilot is capable of organizing his or her own perceptions (in essence, creating internal pathways) to adopt any one of the behavior modes described above. Indeed, a theory referred to as the successive organization of perceptions theory has been forwarded to describe this type of skill development.[44] There appear to be distinct advantages to the pursuit and precognitive control models in terms of improved pilot-vehicle performance and reduced pilot workload.

Remarks

The modes of possible pilot behavior outlined above would certainly appear to complicate the issue of pilot-vehicle analysis. Each of the three pilot-modeling approaches (crossover, synchronous, and OCM) is capable of describing at least the compensatory and pursuit behavior modes.[44] Pilots may trigger APC events by switching from one mode to another (e.g., from pursuit to compensatory control) if the underlying conditions for an APC event are present.

Applying Pilot Models to the APC Problem

If the crossover, synchronous, and OCM pilot models are indeed descriptive of human pilot behavior, the question naturally arises as to whether they can successfully describe conditions that lead to or catalyze PIO problems. Generally speaking, the answer to this question is "yes" for fully developed PIOs. A study by McRuer includes historical background to the successes that have been achieved in this area.[42] Unfortunately, existing pilot models are not suitable for describing the transients of APC phenomena, including the developmental details of non-oscillatory APCs and the initial transient pilot changes involved in Category III PIOs.

6

Criteria for Assessing Aircraft-Pilot Coupling Potential

This chapter examines the status of existing and proposed criteria for assessing APC potential. For fixed-wing aircraft with modest stability augmentation and conventional, fully powered surface actuating systems, Category I PIO tendencies are arguably reduced to a negligible level for aircraft that meet the flying qualities requirements in MIL-F-8785C[69] or that are included in the newer MIL-STD-1797A.[70] Rotorcraft that meet the requirements of ADS-33D[68] should also be resistant to APC events. These flying qualities requirements have been developed over a long period of time using ground and in-flight simulators and experimental, prototype, and operational aircraft. Aircraft parameters and parameter combinations that are sensitive indicators of PIO tendencies have been identified. In addition, pilot assessments that include potential for PIO as a key factor, such as the CH PR (Cooper Harper pilot rating) and PIOR (PIO rating) have been used in empirical studies. In other words, the likelihood of severe Category I PIOs is greatly reduced in aircraft with Level 1 flying qualities. However, Category II and III PIOs are not well covered in these military specifications. Further, the FAA has no equivalent requirements for PIOs of any category.

The control-system characteristics of modern aircraft equipped with FBW FCSs do not necessarily correspond to those of mechanical systems in every detail. Designers have considerable latitude to provide effective aircraft dynamics that are better in some respects than conventional features. Thus classical criteria may not necessarily apply directly to these designs. Perhaps criteria suitable for these configurations need to be substituted for the older criteria that may no longer apply. Or perhaps, to the extent that the specific dynamic properties of a modern aircraft are similar to those of earlier aircraft, PIO-specific criteria should complement existing requirements. Design flexibility and features intrinsic to FBW technology allow—and may require—additional criteria for aspects of the FCS that are markedly different from conventional systems. As some of the more recent events attest, PIOs involving FBW aircraft are not confined to Category I.

This chapter begins with a discussion of the desirable features of APC criteria (i.e., some general prerequisites), providing a rationale for comparing existing and new criteria. Short reviews are then presented of some noteworthy candidate criteria that have been suggested recently.

Existing criteria have focused on PIOs much more than non-oscillatory APC events. Therefore, some serious non-oscillatory APC events that may be involved in closed-loop system divergences have not received in-depth consideration. In the vast majority of severe PIOs, attitude oscillations have been the dominant feature, although both linear and angular accelerations and other cues have also been identified as contributors in some cases. Indeed, the sometimes ambiguous record of predicting PIOs using fixed-base simulators is often cited as indirect evidence that acceleration cues are more important than had been thought. But even in most of the flight research that specifically addresses PIOs in detail, attitude has been considered the predominant cue.[5] Some notable attempts have been made to include criteria involving path and acceleration cues as add-ons to a baseline in which attitude is dominant.[48,66] As might be expected in an empirically based engineering discipline, a great deal of art is needed to cover many situations.[48]

A proper synthesis that includes the above factors cannot be formulated using currently available data and theory. In any event, such a synthesis would greatly exceed the scope of this study. Because attitude control remains at the core of PIO problems, either in its own right or as a key inner-loop constituent, and because most research has been devoted to attitude control, this assessment of APC criteria is focused on oscillatory APC events involving pitch and roll attitude control problems.

To meet the needs of the several technical communities concerned with these issues, the following reviews are presented in two parts: general overviews and more detailed treatments of topics of interest primarily to specialists. The more specialized segments include elementary quantitative examples in which the criterion under discussion is applied to an idealized simple effective aircraft. The same effective aircraft example is used for each criteria discussed, thereby providing a basis for comparisons.

Essentially all of the reviews specifically address Category I PIOs, as there are no general criteria for Category II and III APC events. However, some analytical procedures for Categories II and III do exist, and some recent developments that show promise for predicting Category II conditions primarily associated with rate limiting are described at the end of this chapter.

PREREQUISITES FOR CRITERIA

A useful criterion must satisfy three prerequisites: validity, selectivity, and ready applicability.

Validity

"Validity" implies that a criterion embodies properties and characteristics that define the environment of interest and are associated with parameter spaces covering the vast majority of known cases. Because the PVS is a central component in severe PIOs, the criterion must relate to closed-loop, high-gain, aggressive, urgent, and precise piloted-control behavior. The connection can be either explicit or implicit; but it must derive from and reflect, in some sense, the fundamental principle that pilot actions combine with aircraft actions to result in a PIO. At a subtler level, it must be kept in mind that these combinations seldom occur, so the criterion should also emphasize the rarity of the events.

A logical assumption is that effective aircraft dynamics are designed to provide good flying qualities during normal flight maneuvers and tasks. The term good flying qualities includes very small, high-frequency effective time lags that do not require pilot compensation under normal circumstances and other features that are directly associated with exceptional pilot-aircraft properties in high-gain tracking-like situations. To be valid, the parameters in a criterion should somehow reflect these features.

The rarity of severe PIOs may also reflect the rarity of triggering events (i.e., out-of-the-norm, system-forcing functions or disturbances). Thus, a criterion that may guard against PIOs during normal maneuvers and small inputs may be useful even if it does not focus on flying qualities cliffs under extreme or unusual circumstances. Such a criterion would be valid for Category I events but could not rule out Category II or III tendencies.

The most useful criteria, of course, will give more information than simple pass/fail results. They will also provide additional information, such as relevance to specific PIO categories, conditions of validity (hence giving some hints about situations of unassessed risk), and frequency and bounding amplitudes of oscillation (which may indicate potential severity). Simple pass/fail results for a set of definable, likely circumstances are useful starting points. As a minimum, a "fail" can be a warning, and a "pass" can provide clearance with respect to a restricted group of APC possibilities. An explicit reference to the circumstances of a pass/fail result may indicate some of the more detailed, descriptive features that should be further examined by applying the analysis and simulation procedures described in Chapter 5.

Selectivity

"Selectivity" demands that the criterion differentiate sharply between "good" and "bad" systems. Criteria that downgrade the performance of aircraft that are actually adequate may be too restrictive. But there should be a clear differentiation at the level of acceptability. In the context of PIO prediction, the most important selectivity feature is the capability of distinguishing configurations that may be susceptible to *severe* PIOs from those that are not.

Ready Applicability

"Ready applicability" requires that the criterion be easily and conveniently applied. Expression of the criterion in terms of readily available system parameters should be compact. Procedures for analytical evaluations using the criterion should be convenient. The criterion measures should be easily determined using analytical models and/or empirical methods involving simulations or the actual aircraft and its systems.

PROMINENT ASSESSMENT CRITERIA FOR CATEGORY I

The most prominent criteria or partial criteria that have been proposed for assessing attitude-dominant Category I PIOs are the following:

- Aircraft-Bandwidth/Phase Delay, ω_{BW} and τ_p [48,49]
- Gain/Phase Template, including ω_{180}/Average Phase Rate[8,22,24]
- Smith-Geddes Attitude-Dominant Type III[64,66]
- Neal-Smith (original version,[53] updated version,[70] Moscow Aviation Institute version[18])
- Dropback[21,22]

The theoretical bases for these criteria can all be related to a closed-loop PVS. Smith-Geddes Type III and Neal-Smith are explicitly based on pilot models related to compensatory control. The others are more implicitly connected with closed-loop piloting activities. The Aircraft-Bandwidth/Phase Delay and ω_{180}/Average Phase Rate boundary constructions occupy a middle ground in that they reflect effective aircraft properties that affect high-gain, closed-loop control. Dropback measures are, strictly speaking, open-loop transient response properties of the aircraft, so their connection with closed-loop operations is the most obscure of this set of criteria. Nevertheless, a subtle connection does exist.

The Gain/Phase Templates, including ω_{180}/Average Phase Rate boundaries, consider the effective aircraft attitude dynamics as an element of an open-loop system exhibited as coordinates on a gain/phase chart. (This and the other criteria forms are illustrated below in connection with their short reviews.) These open-loop effective aircraft characteristics can be explicitly associated with closed-loop PVS operations in which the pilot's behavior is synchronous (pure gain). The Aircraft-Bandwidth/Phase Delay measures are vehicle properties chosen to reflect key aspects of vehicle dynamics that affect the ease of pilot control and the tolerance for pilot dynamic variations in the crossover frequency region of the PVS during high-gain, precision-control activities.

The various parameters or metrics in all these criteria are typically used as coordinates to define parameter spaces. Boundaries in terms of these parameters are established to encompass pilot-rating data appropriate to given flying qualities levels or other concerns based on pilot ratings. Because pilot ratings are sensitive measures of the dynamics a pilot must exhibit to exert appropriate control in closed-loop tasks, the ratings intrinsically reflect both pilot and vehicle dynamics. The actual boundary lines for a given parameter, such as oscillatory APC potential or flying qualities levels, can then be drawn to reflect the desired qualities.

In principle, the boundaries could be different for different closed-loop task scenarios (e.g., precision tracking and tight regulation, closed-loop maneuvers, and large-amplitude corrective maneuvers) and for different types of pilot behavior. The boundaries for rotorcraft are a case in point.[68] For fixed-wing aircraft, the boundaries for Neal-Smith, Aircraft-Bandwidth/Phase Delay, Gain/Phase Template, ω_{180}/Average Phase Rate, and Dropback criteria have traditionally been drawn to distinguish between flying qualities Levels 1, 2, and 3. Only recently has considerable attention been given to boundaries peculiarly sensitive to PIO potential.

The following summary is provided for readers who are not concerned with the details and rationale for individual criteria. When viewed from an appropriate perspective, all the PIO assessment criteria for Category I PIOs listed above can provide insights and data that are useful in understanding PIO situations and their likelihood. At the moment, no one criterion meets all three prerequisites for criteria or delivers all the desired information—that is, none provides a comprehensive pass/fail estimate in terms of the frequency and circumstances of PIO occurrence. (PIO amplitude must be added for Category II and III situations.)

Each of the five criteria listed above is described below, followed by a discussion of extending these criteria to the lateral axis. In addition, a discussion on estimating the frequency of Category I oscillatory APC events is interposed between the discussions of the Smith-Geddes and Neal-Smith criteria.

$$\tau_p = \frac{\Delta\phi\, 2\omega_{180}}{57.3\,(2\omega_{180})}$$

Rate response-types: ω_{BW} is lesser of $\omega_{BW_{gain}}$ and $\omega_{BW_{phase}}$

Attitude response-types: $\omega_{BW} = \omega_{BW_{phase}}$

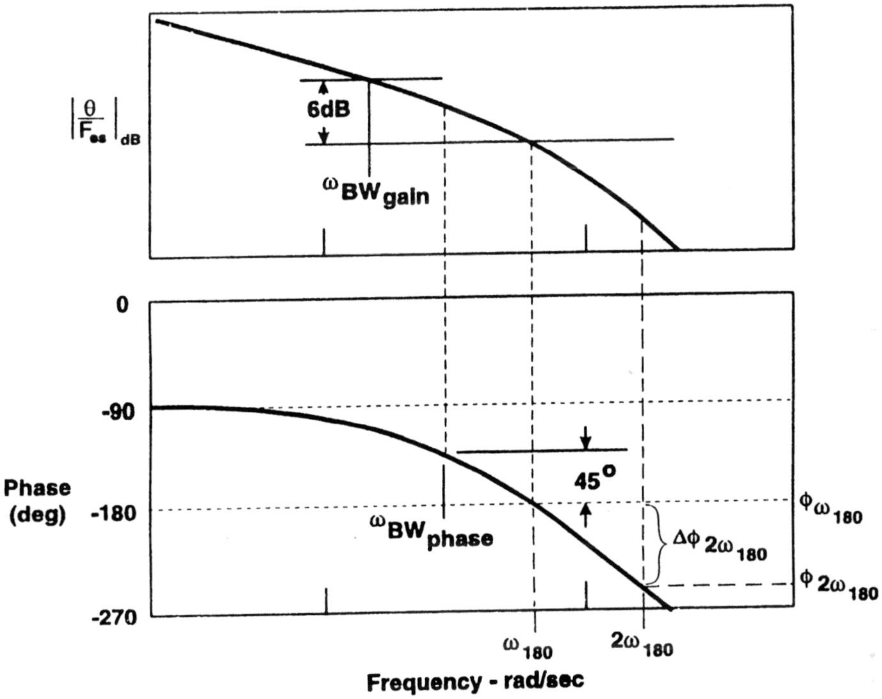

FIGURE 6-1 Definitions of aircraft pitch attitude bandwidth and phase delay. Source: Adapted from Mitchell et al.[49]

Aircraft-Bandwidth/Phase Delay

Aircraft-Bandwidth and Phase Delay are popular and effective criteria measures that have been successfully used to evaluate flying qualities.[48,49] As illustrated in Figure 6-1, these are frequency-domain metrics that focus on particular characteristics of the aircraft attitude transfer function. The aircraft-attitude bandwidth, ω_{BW}, is a measure of the range of frequencies over which a pilot can exert good closed-loop control without having to compensate excessively (e.g., through the development of phase lead or the anticipation needed to offset the time lags in effective aircraft dynamics). The aircraft-attitude bandwidth is also a measure of the range of frequencies within which the aircraft dynamics can accommodate changes in pilot gain that are necessary to execute both moderately and highly demanding tasks.

The phase delay, τ_p, limits the attainable closed-loop PVS bandwidth and governs the sensitivity to pilot gain of the PVS closed-loop resonance characteristics when the PVS is operating at the highest gains. The term "phase delay" is sometimes confusing because its dimensions are in seconds, but it is also an indication of the initial time delay in a response to pilot step inputs. Thus it is, at least partly, a time-domain measure.

Because these metrics are intimately related to closed-loop pilot-vehicle control and because they support a parameter space that covers almost all known cases, they satisfy the validity criterion.[48] That is, within the frequency band defined by appropriate values of the aircraft bandwidth and phase delay, the effective aircraft dynamics tolerate either high or low pilot-gain and demand very little lead or other pilot compensation. They also satisfy the ready-applicability criterion in that they are ordinarily easy to extrapolate from analyses, simulations, flight test data, etc.

A useful indication of PVS sensitivity to gain changes near instability, when viewed in gain/phase coordinates, is the slope of the gain-phase curve in that region. Gibson[24] defines Average Phase Rate as follows:

$$\text{Average Phase Rate, } \phi'_{\omega u} = (\phi_{\omega_{180}} - \phi_{2\omega_{180}}) / \omega_{180} \quad \text{(Equation 6-1)}$$

This slope is usually expressed in degrees/Hz.

A comparison with Figure 6-1 shows that the average phase rate and the phase delay are directly related. In general, the average phase rate is 720 τ_p degrees/Hz. Because the average phase rate is a direct multiple of the phase delay, it can be treated here along with the phase delay. It is a primary PIO indicator in the Gain/Phase Template, including ω_{180}/Average Phase Rate criterion, which will be discussed next.

For single-loop PVSs, an idealized controlled element transfer function is $Y_c = K_c/s$. Here, Y_c is the transfer function that operates on the pilot's output to produce the system response, K_c is the controlled element gain, and the 1/s indicates an integration. As an idealization of longitudinal or lateral axis dynamics, this rate-control transfer characteristic results in constant-velocity pitching or rolling responses to pilot-imposed step-function command inputs to the elevators or ailerons. This characteristic also results in steady-state changes in pitch or bank angle in response to pulse inputs from the inceptors. For nonpilots, the characteristic can be envisioned as the idealized directional dynamics of a car when the turn rate is directly proportional to the deflection of the steering wheel.

These time-response attributes are the open-loop, effective aircraft properties. They are favorable for closed-loop piloted control because the pilot can close the loop acting in a pure-gain fashion in which pilot output is proportional to perceived error. There is thus no need for the pilot to generate any lead (anticipation) or lag compensation to close the loop. Furthermore, these idealized vehicle dynamics permit a very large range of pilot-gain adjustments. By simply increasing or decreasing gain, the pilot can establish a very wide range of closed-loop PVS bandwidths for the desired level of control precision without compromising the stability of the closed-loop system.

In terms of the open-loop PVS, gain changes directly change the open-loop crossover frequency. In the frequency domain, this ideal aircraft has an infinite aircraft-bandwidth, ω_{BW}, and zero phase delay. Features such as the PVS open-loop crossover frequency, precision of control, and disturbance suppression are totally controlled by the gain adopted by the pilot. With these idealized effective aircraft dynamics, the pilot's lags become the limiting factor in closed-loop operations. The closed-loop neutral stability frequency for this PVS, when pilot lags are taken into account, is 0.84 Hz (5.25 rad/sec); this frequency can be considered to be at or near the upper limit for closed-loop compensatory control.[42]

Well-designed aircraft and FCSs can produce attitude characteristics in the effective aircraft dynamics that approximate the ideal K_c/s form in the region of PVS crossover, thereby requiring very little pilot lead and permitting large variations in pilot gain. The higher-frequency effective aircraft dynamics, however, contribute a variety of lags and leads that alter the (stability-constrained) available crossover region both quantitatively and qualitatively. These higher frequency dynamics have a first-order effect on the aircraft-attitude bandwidth, ω_{BW}, which for "good" aircraft can be measured by the frequency at which $\angle Y_c = -135$ degrees. This corresponds to a pure-gain pilot loop-closure with a phase margin of 45 degrees (i.e., 180 degrees minus 135 degrees). A phase margin of zero corresponds to a PIO of the PVS. The change in closed-loop system resonance (i.e., peak magnification ratio*) as a result of a change in pilot gain is governed by how fast the phase is changing at frequencies somewhat higher than the aircraft bandwidth frequency. Thus, a phase that changes slowly at frequencies above ω_{BW} permits a larger, smoother, and better graded increase in pilot gain without undue changes in the closed-loop system characteristics than is possible with a more rapidly changing phase. The pilot is confronted with a less drastic change in closed-loop system properties when operating near the maximum gain levels.

At the limits of control encountered with high pilot gains, where the phase effects are significant, the aircraft bandwidth alone is not a sufficient measure. The phase delay (τ_p) accounts for these higher-frequency features.[49] As a closed-loop system metric, the phase delay emphasizes the aircraft contribution to the phase changes in the region of the unstable frequency for

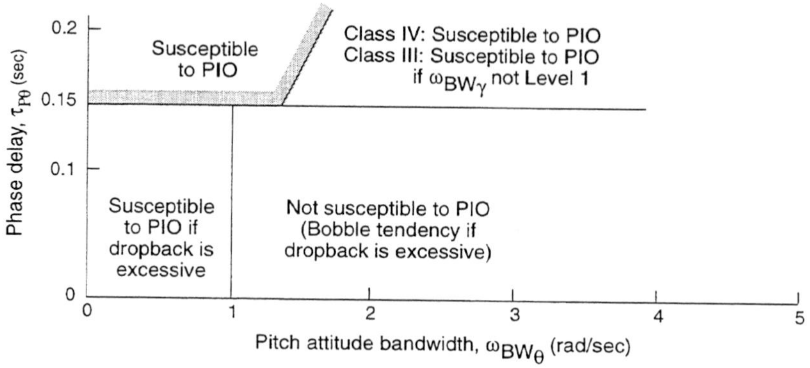

FIGURE 6-2 Aircraft-Bandwidth/Phase Delay/Dropback requirements for PIO resistance in terminal flight phases. Source: Klyde.[39]

the effective PVS. When the pilot is operating in a pure gain (i.e., synchronous) mode, this is the total system phase change. Therefore, it should be particularly sensitive to synchronous-pilot Category I PIOs, although it is not confined to this variety.

The particular boundaries in the Airplane Bandwidth/Phase Delay space can be drawn to include or exclude data points in the experimental pilot ratings and other PVS data. Thus, when boundaries connected with flying qualities levels are appropriate, the critical data sets may include high-gain tracking tasks (where the compensatory control and pursuit modes of pilot behavior are important), as well as precision maneuvers (where combined open-loop and closed-loop pilot operations are important, i.e., where pursuit and precognitive control modes may be major discriminators).

For PIOs, data sets appropriate for either or both compensatory and synchronous high-pilot-gain operations are relevant. PIO-specific boundaries would incorporate Level 1 flying qualities boundaries as a subset because a PIO-prone aircraft can never be considered to have Level 1 flying qualities. (Level 1 flying qualities are defined as "clearly adequate for the mission . . . aircraft is satisfactory without improvement."[20])

Bandwidth and phase delay boundaries pertinent to predicting PIOs that take into account data from research aircraft have been used to examine in detail the application of bandwidth and phase delay concepts to Category I PIO assessment. These boundaries are, of course, tuned and refined as the data base expands. The boundaries shown in Figure 6-2 are the best and most current. Aircraft-Bandwidth/Phase Delay criteria boundaries are "most effective at correlating PIO tendency ratings for pitch tracking and landing."[70] The region not susceptible to PIO is the rectangle defined by $1 \leq \omega_{BW} \leq 6$ rad/sec and $0 \leq \tau_p \leq 0.15$. Other considerations, such as dropback, can be used to expand the PIO-prone space on an ad hoc basis.[48]

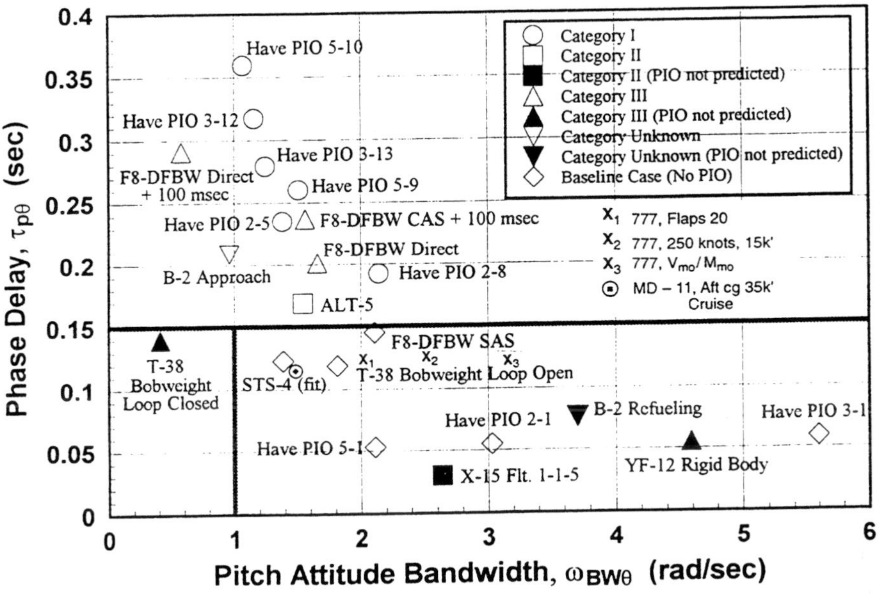

FIGURE 6-3 Aircraft-Bandwidth/Phase Delay parameters as indicators of PIO susceptibility for sample operational and test aircraft. Source: Adapted from Klyde.[39]

In Figure 6-3, a variety of operational and test aircraft are plotted against these basic boundaries. The results show that the boundaries are generally very good for distinguishing between severe PIOs of the Have PIO configurations and their non-PIO baseline conditions (i.e., Have PIO configurations 2-1, 3-1, and 5-1).[5] (Have PIO refers to a series of experiments that collected important PIO data during flight experiments with aircraft in various configurations. Indeed, these data had much to do with establishing the boundaries). The ALT-5 case is shown as PIO prone, although it is close to the upper boundary of non-PIO prone configurations. The F-8 DFBW PIO case can be traced through various sequences from CAS + 100 ms to Direct + 100 ms to Direct to SAS. The highest quality and most complete data enclosed by the boundaries are consistent with pilot operations in a compensatory context, so the boundaries are certainly pertinent for these situations. Synchronous-pilot data points may also be included.

The very limited Category II and III situations (e.g., PIOs for aircraft such as YF-12 and X-15) are generally not well covered by the Aircraft-Bandwidth/Phase Delay boundaries per se. The linear manifestations of these tendencies occur well within the "not susceptible" region. The addition of an "excessive dropback" region permits the inclusion of the T-38 PIO, during which the pilot behavior was almost surely synchronous.

One problem with the application of Aircraft-Bandwidth/Phase Delay criteria is the definition of the input to the effective aircraft. As currently defined, input is inceptor force (although for much of the data underlying the criterion, position could be used just as well).[48] Thus, lags and nonlinearities in the artificial feel system are explicitly included in measurements of attitude/control input transfer characteristics. On FBW aircraft, the nature of the pilot's inceptor can be more varied than on conventional aircraft, ranging from force sticks to driven columns with proprioceptive display features, such as force changes feeding back various pieces of information. The pilot's limb-neuromuscular system (i.e., the pilot's "actuation elements") can accommodate a wide variety of feel-system nonlinear characteristics.[27] Consequently, it may not be reasonable to confine the form of pilot input.

In applying the Aircraft-Bandwidth/Phase Delay and other frequency domain criteria to the Boeing 777, a distinct preference was developed for inceptor position because "position-based data yield more consistent and coherent frequency response results and reduce uncertainty in determination of phase delay and bandwidth.[54] Boeing also found that using position inputs simplified comparisons of feel-system frequency responses for all their aircraft.

In general, the data base on transport aircraft in terms of Aircraft-Bandwidth/Phase Delay and Average Phase Rate is small. It has been significantly expanded during the course of this study by Boeing's release of flight data for several aircraft.[54] These data demonstrate that the 747, 757, 767-300ER, and the 777 (in "normal," "secondary," and "direct" FCS modes) have phase delay values of less than 0.14 sec when column position is used as the input. The aircraft attitude bandwidth values also fall within the Figure 6-3 boundaries. Specific examples for the 777 based on in-flight measurements are included in Figure 6-3. Another example is shown for the MD-11 using estimates with $\tau_{p\theta}$ values based on column deflection rather than column force. Thus the boundaries of Figure 6-3 for attitude-dominant PIOs, which were originally based primarily on data from fighter and research aircraft, appear to be applicable to transport aircraft as long as input is appropriately identified.

The Aircraft-Bandwidth/Phase Delay indicators do not explicitly estimate likely PIO frequency. However, the synchronous-pilot ($Y_p = K_p$) PVS neutral stability frequency ($\omega_u = \omega_{180}$) is used in the calculation of the phase delay, although this frequency is not always called out as part of the PIO assessment information. When it is called out, and to the extent that PIOs are associated with open-loop pilot characteristics that approximate a pure gain at the PIO frequency, ω_{180} is an estimate for ω_{PIO}. But, to the extent that the PIO is a phenomenon of a compensatory PVS, ω_{180} can be an incorrect estimate. It is important to note that this discussion of PIO frequency estimates does not imply that the suggested Aircraft-Bandwidth/Phase Delay boundaries for PIO shown in Figures 6-2 and 6-3 assume synchronous-pilot control behavior.

For most extended-rigid-body effective aircraft dynamics, where the higher frequency flexible modes do not significantly affect the phase or amplitude ratio* plots at frequencies below or near 2 ω_{180}, the bandwidth and phase delay measurements are usually straightforward. These measures could be more ambiguous in situations of roll-attitude control if lateral-directional coupling effects are prominent near ω_{BW}, ω_{180}, or 2 ω_{180}. Uncertainties and ambiguities also appear in the presence of flexible-body modes, as in the case of the YF-12.

Illustrative Example

To illustrate the use of Aircraft-Bandwidth/Phase Delay and Average Phase Rate for predicting severe APC events, consider that the controlled element attitude dynamics can be approximated in the region of the PVS crossover frequency by the transfer function:

$$Y_c = \frac{K_c e^{-j\omega\tau_c}}{j\omega} \qquad \text{(Equation 6-2)}$$

This simple, idealized form is an appropriate first-order approximation of the attitude properties in the crossover frequency region for well designed effective aircraft dynamics. It is worth emphasizing again that this elementary form is intended to approximate a restricted range of frequencies and that the effective time delay (τ_e) is a composite low-frequency approximation to a potentially large number of lead and lag time constants and pure time delays that may occur well above the crossover frequency region.

The open-loop Bode diagrams* (i.e., gain and phase versus frequency) and gain/phase diagrams for this system are shown in Figure 6-4. On the gain/phase plot, the gain (K_c) is arbitrarily set so that the crossover frequency (where the amplitude ratio is 1.0 or 0 dB) occurs when the phase is -110 degrees, to be consistent with the convention adopted by Buchacker, et al,. for gain/phase templates.[8] The aircraft bandwidth (ω_{BW}) and the instability frequency ($\omega_u = \omega_{180}$) for a pure-gain closure are identified on the figure. For this system, the quantities are given by $\omega_{BW} = \pi/4\tau_e$ rad/sec [$f_{BW} = 1/8\tau_e$ Hz], and $\omega_u = \pi/2\tau_e$ [$f_u = 1/4\tau_e$ Hz]. The phase delay for this effective controlled element is $\tau_p = \tau_e/2$. The average phase rate (ϕ_{ω_u}) is a direct multiple of the phase delay (by 720 degree/Hz), so it will be 320 τ_e degree/Hz.

Table 6-1 shows aircraft bandwidth, phase delay, and average phase rate characteristics for a sequence of τ_e values for this idealized rate-command-controlled element. It also shows the neutral stability frequency when the system is closed by a synchronous pilot.

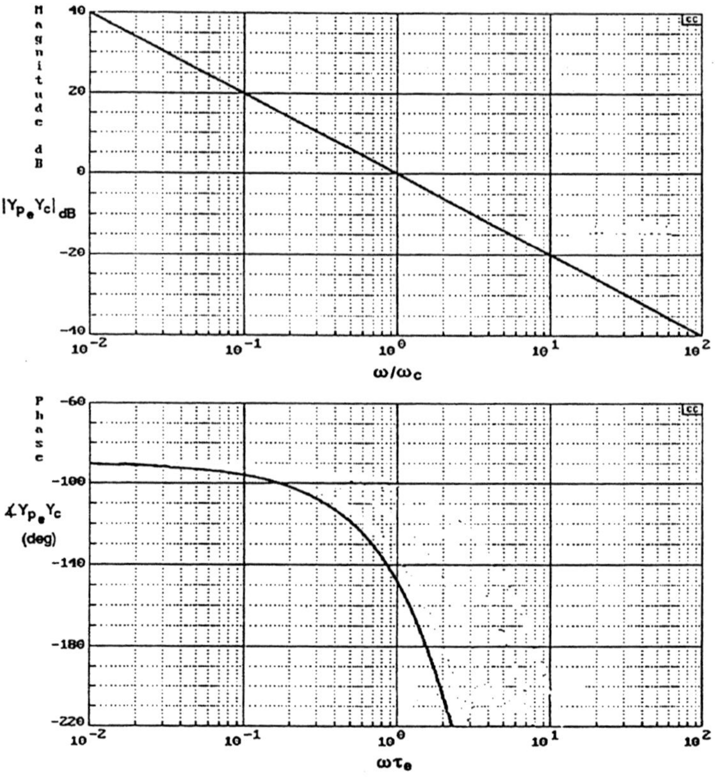

Bode Diagrams

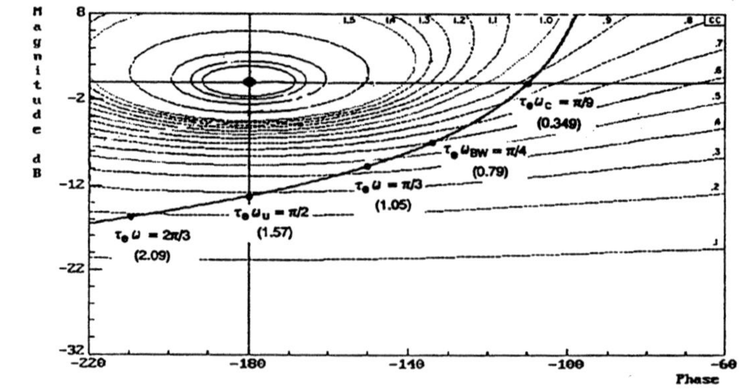

Gain Phase Diagram

FIGURE 6-4 Bode and gain phase diagram presentations for $K_c e^{-s\tau}/s$. Source: Klyde.[39]

TABLE 6-1 Idealized Rate-Command Controlled Element Characteristics

τ_e (sec)	ω_{BW_θ} (rad/sec)	τ_{p_θ} (sec)	ω_u (rad/sec)	f_{180} (Hz)	ϕ_{ω_u} (deg/rad/sec)	(deg/Hz)
0.10	7.85	0.05	15.7	2.5	5.73	36
0.15	5.24	0.075	10.5	1.67	8.60	54
0.20	3.93	0.10	7.85	1.25	11.46	72
0.25	3.14	0.125	6.28	1.0	14.32	90
↓ PIO potential for Aircraft-Bandwidth/Phase Delay						
0.30	2.62	0.15	5.23	0.83	17.19	108
0.35	2.24	0.175	4.49	0.71	20.06	126
				↓ PIO potential for ω_{180}/Average Phase Rate		
0.40	1.96	0.20	3.92	0.62	22.92	144
0.45	1.75	0.225	3.49	0.55	25.78	162
0.50	1.57	0.25	3.14	0.50	28.65	180

Source: McRuer.[42]

The Aircraft-Bandwidth/Phase Delay boundaries in Figure 6-2 suggest that an aircraft will be susceptible to PIOs if $\tau_p \geq 0.15$ sec for Flight Phase Categories B and C.[48] (Note that these categories refer to flight phases rather than to PIO categories. Flight Phase Categories are part of the flying qualities esoterica—Flight Phase Category C, for instance, refers to terminal flight phases including approach and landing.) Thus, statements in the study by Mitchell, et al., are compatible for Flight Phase Categories B and C. For Flight Phase Category A (nonterminal flight phases that require rapid maneuvering, precision tracking, or precise flight-path control), $\tau_p \geq 0.19$ is unfavorable from a PIO standpoint.[48] In terms of the Table 6-1 cases, these criteria would imply that idealized rate-command effective vehicle characteristics with effective time delay parameters greater than 0.38 sec for Category A flight or 0.30 sec for Categories B and C are likely to be prone to PIO.

This example will be used again to illustrate other candidate criteria.

Gain/Phase Template (including ω_{180}/Average Phase Rate) Criteria

The Gain/Phase Template (including ω_{180}/Average Phase Rate Criteria) has some of the same features as the Aircraft-Bandwidth/Phase Delay criteria, with an additional element for the gain of the effective aircraft dynamics.[24] The criteria are shown in Figure 6-5. The boundaries, which are defined in terms of the frequency at 180-degree phase lag of the pitch attitude frequency response, ω_{180}, and the average phase rate, are similar in form to the Aircraft-Bandwidth/Phase Delay plot of Figure 6-3, except for the details. If synchronous-pilot activity is assumed, this formulation directly indicates the PIO frequency region.

The boundaries in Figure 6-5 were originally intended to indicate flying qualities in general rather than PIOs in particular. A comparison of Figures 6-3 and 6-5 shows that flight data (such as Have PIO 2-8) fall along the L2-L3 boundary.[5] This boundary is currently used as a dividing line for assessing PIO potential. In drawing this boundary, Gibson intended that it discriminate, among other things, between PIO-prone and non-PIO cases with which he was familiar. It does accomplish this for much of the data shown in Figure 6-3. Like other proposed boundaries, however, this one is subject to adjustment and fine tuning as more data become available.

Note that the average phase rate associated with PIO-prone conditions would correspond to a phase delay of 0.20 sec. This is 0.05 sec larger than the phase delay in Figure 6-3 but very close to the 0.19 sec suggested for Flight Phase Category A. Thus, in Table 6-1, the PIO potential dividing line based on the average phase rate from Figure 6-5 is at a lower level for the idealized rate-command controlled element than the dividing line based on Figure 6-3.

A notable difference between the Gain/Phase Template and other criteria reviewed here is the attempt to quantify the gain of the effective aircraft dynamics. This is shown in the amplitude boundaries portion of Figure 6-5. The boundaries are based on center stick inceptors as the cockpit longitudinal control devices. Analogous values for other inceptors have not yet been established.

Smith-Geddes Attitude-Dominant Type III Criterion

The application of the Smith-Geddes criterion for attitude-dominant PIOs has been developed and described.[64,66] As the basis for this criterion, Smith developed a very simple linear formula for the crossover frequency from an early (circa 1965) series of extensive, fixed-base experiments on a cross section of elementary systems. The formula is

$$\omega_c = 6.0 + 0.24m \qquad \text{(Equation 6-3)}$$

where m is an "average slope" in dB/octave of the effective aircraft dynamics in the crossover region.[64] This formula does not explicitly depend on the phase rate It provides an estimate of the crossover frequency for a compensatory PVS based on controlled element dynamics other than the dynamics on which the equation is based.

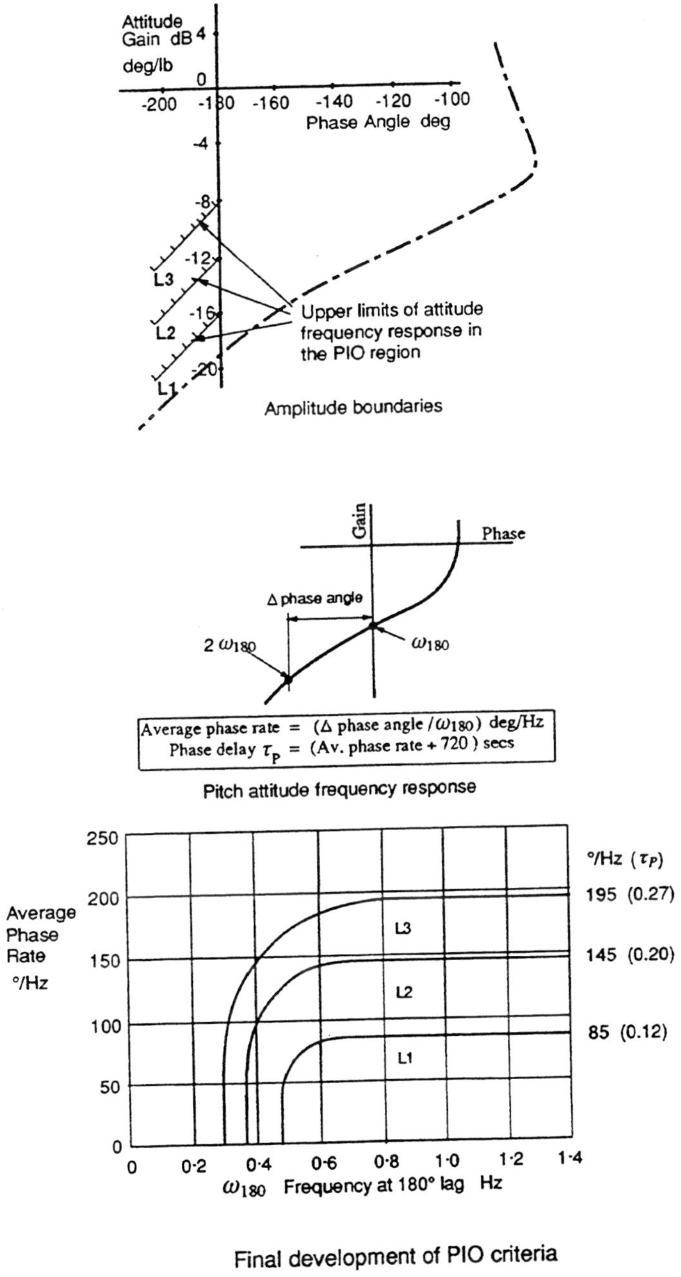

FIGURE 6-5 Gain/Phase Template, ω_{180}/Average Phase Rate Boundaries. Source: Gibson.[24]

The elementary system dynamics ($Y_c = K_c$, K_c /s, and K_c /s^2) used to develop the empirical data base had no higher-frequency net lags. The pilot's inceptor was a spring-restrained side stick with no other dynamics, and all measurements were based on stick position (although the spring restraint was linear, so the pilot's output force is proportional to the stick deflection). Therefore, this crossover frequency is appropriate to the crossover model for conditions where high-frequency lags and leads beyond the crossover region are not included; aircraft lags within the crossover region are implicitly included.[45] (In this context, the crossover region, would extend from about 1 to 8 rad/sec [0.16 to 1.27 Hz].) When the lags associated with more complex effective aircraft dynamics are included, the nominally positive phase margins associated with the elementary system types on which the formula is based may be assumed if the same crossover characteristics are maintained.

The Smith-Geddes Type III criterion for attitude-dominant PIOs is a straightforward test of whether or not a positive phase margin exists when the actual effective aircraft dynamics are examined at the crossover frequency. That is, an attitude-dominant, compensatory system, single-loop PIO is predicted if the following condition is met:

$$\angle \theta / F_{es} (j\omega_c) \leq -180 \text{ degrees} \qquad \text{(Equation 6-4)}$$

Although this criterion explicitly involves only the effective aircraft dynamics, θ/F_{es}, relating the pitch attitude to the stick force, the pilot characteristics have been accounted for via the definition of the crossover frequency, which is also referred to as the criterion frequency.

As a PIO predictor, the Smith-Geddes Type III criterion works well for Category I severe PIOs (which are essentially linear) from the Have PIO data.[5] The criterion is selective between "good" baselines and severe PIO subsets. It has accurately predicted that a variety of aircraft were prone to PIO.[64] The criterion was also effective in showing PIO tendencies for configurations in the data base compiled by Neal and Smith (1970).[53]

The ω_c column in Table 6-2 is based on the Smith-Geddes Type III formula, while ω_{PIO} and $\phi(\theta/F_{es})$ are measured data for the operational and test aircraft documented in the study by Klyde et al.,[39] and the severe PIOs from the Have PIO data base.[5] The PIO Prone column is based on the Smith-Geddes Type III criterion. As shown in Table 6-2, the Shuttle ALT-5, F-8 DFBW, and Have PIO data are well covered by the Smith-Geddes criterion.

The Smith-Geddes Type III criterion has been proposed for addition to the MIL-STD-1797A along with features of the Gain/Phase Template.[70] The review of research aircraft data gathered after the original development of handling quality requirements for the design of the fighter aircraft[48,66] indicates that the Smith-Geddes criterion can be very conservative; that is, it may predict that more configurations are susceptible to PIOs than actually are.

TABLE 6-2 Prediction of PIO Susceptibility with Smith-Geddes Attitude-Dominant Type III Criterion for Operational and Test Aircraft

Aircraft	ω_{PIO} (rad/sec)	ω_c (rad/sec)	$\phi(\theta/F_{es})$ (deg)	Type III PIO Prone
Have PIO 2-1 (baseline)	no PIO	4.37	-161.0	no
Have PIO 2-5	2.7	3.18	-211.6	yes
Have PIO 2-8	3.8	4.33	-201.5	yes
Have PIO 3-1 (baseline)	no PIO	5.06	-127.9	no
Have PIO 3-12	2.2	3.26	-225.6	yes
Have PIO 3-13	3.2	3.97	-223.9	yes
Have PIO 5-1 (baseline)	no PIO	3.77	-167.6	no
Have PIO 5-9	3.5	3.56	-216.9	yes
Have PIO 5-10	2.7	3.14	-229.5	yes
X-15 Flight 1-1-5	3.3	4.14	-170.9	no
T-38 Bobweight Closed	7.8	5.52	-66.0	no
T-38 Bobweight Open	7.8	5.45	-108.4	no
YF-12 Rigid Body Only	3.5	4.97	-142.6	no
Shuttle ALT-5	3.4	3.84	-193.1	yes
F-8 DFBW CAS + 100 msec	3.1	4.10	-215.2	yes
F-8 DFBW Direct + 100 msec	3.1	3.65	-232.5	yes
F-8 DFBW Direct	3.1	3.65	-211.6	yes
F-8 DFBW SAS	3.1	4.15	-179.8	borderline
B-2 Off-Nominal Approach	2.7	3.21	-210.0	yes
B-2 Aerial Refueling	3.8	5.05	-158.0	no

Source: Klyde.[39]

Of the 51 cases examined by Mitchell et al,[48] the Smith-Geddes criterion predicted that 48 should be susceptible to PIO, but only 17 actually exhibited PIOs. All configurations with a PIOR of 3 or greater were in the latter group, whereas many of the configurations with PIORs of 1 did not exhibit PIO tendencies.

The Smith-Geddes Type III criterion was used to evaluate a variety of Boeing aircraft (757-200, 767-300ER, 747-400, and 777). All passed the criterion, although several were marginal (6 data points out of 15 had phase angles ranging from –165 to –180 degrees at the criterion frequency; only 1 point was from a 777)[54] The frequency response data was based on column position as an input. The 6 data points of highest quality in this set were for the 777 (in "normal," "secondary," and "direct" FCS modes) engaged in very high gain, simulated, aerial refueling tasks. It received a CH PR of 2 and a PIOR of 1 to 2 from both evaluating pilots.

Illustrative Example

When the Smith-Geddes criterion is applied to the elementary example of an idealized rate-command effective aircraft ($i.e., Y_c = K_c e^{-j\omega\tau_e}/j\omega$), the criterion frequency (ω_c) is,

$$\begin{aligned}\omega_c &= 6.0 + 0.24\ m \qquad \text{(Equation 6-5)}\\ &= 6.0 + 0.24\ (-6\ \text{dB/octave})\\ &= 4.56\ \text{rad/sec}\end{aligned}$$

The effective time delay (τ_e) corresponding to a predicted PIO condition is

$$4.56\tau_e = \frac{\pi}{2},\ \text{or}\ \tau_e = 0.344\ \text{sec} \qquad \text{(Equation 6-6)}$$

This corresponds to a phase delay (τ_p) of 0.172 sec and an average phase rate of 124 deg/Hz. These values are close to the analogous values under the Aircraft-Bandwidth/Phase Delay and Gain/Phase Template, including ω_{180}/Average Phase Rate criteria. The effective time delay is less than the 0.20 sec from the Average Phase Delay criterion and lies midway between the estimates of 0.15 and 0.19 sec from the Aircraft-Bandwidth/Phase Delay boundaries for Flight Phase Category A and Flight Phase Categories B and C.

Comparison of assessments for PIO potential using Gain/Phase Templates, Aircraft-Bandwidth/Phase Delay Criteria, and the Smith-Geddes Type III criterion for this example is somewhat confusing. That is, in this instance Smith-Geddes appears to occupy a middle ground and is not overly conservative. Taking everything into account, one could conclude that meeting the Smith-Geddes Type III criterion indicates a very low probability of an attitude-dominant PIO, although failing it does not necessarily mean that a PIO will occur.

An important aspect of PIO assessment is the estimate of the likely PIO frequency. Using the Smith-Geddes Type III criterion, the criterion frequency of Equation 6-3 is the estimated crossover frequency of the pilot-aircraft open-loop system and also the PIO frequency. The consequences of this can be tested with the Have PIO,[5] which are recapitulated as part of Table 6-2. A linear regression for the six severe PIO cases gives

$$\omega_{PIO} = -0.05 + 0.86\omega_c,\quad r = 0.97 \qquad \text{(Equation 6-7)}$$

The regression is shown in Figure 6-6, which also contains the other data from Table 6-2. In general, Figure 6-6 demonstrates that the estimate of the frequency of Category I PIOs using the existing formula for ω_c is higher than has actually been observed. This implies that the effects of higher frequency lags are underestimated in the Smith-Geddes determination of the criterion frequency. This is surely one reason for the lack of selectivity of the criterion as it is currently constituted.

Equation 6-3 gives a high value for ω_c for a variety of underlying reasons. They include the very high performance levels of the subjects for the experiments (which were conducted 30 years ago) and the very linear, no-lag, side-stick-like inceptor that was used. Equation 6-3 could probably be refined to be more selective using the much more extensive data now available.[45] These data would give less conservative results and could also be adjusted to account for specific inceptor types and experimental scenarios, such as fixed-base, moving-base, or in-flight simulations.

The fundamental Bode relationships between amplitude ratio and phase show that all the minimum-phase properties of a transfer function can be accounted for by defining either the amplitude-ratio or the phase over all frequencies. By including a term involving the amplitude ratio slope in the Equation 6-3 formula for the crossover frequency, the phase lags that have amplitude-ratio effects in the region of the slope measurement are taken into (very) approximate account. But any higher frequency lags from dynamics well above the crossover frequency appear as non-minimum-phase contributions in the frequency range covered by Equation 6-3 and are not reflected in local measurements of the amplitude-ratio slope. There were no such lags in the empirical data on which Equation 6-3 was based. Consequently, adjusting the equation to take into account the higher frequency contributions may be appropriate. The effect would be to reduce the criterion frequency and make the Smith-Geddes Type III estimate of PIO tendencies less conservative.

An important feature of the ready applicability of a criterion is the manner in which the amplitude-ratio slope (m) is computed. Fitting a frequency-response amplitude ratio with a straight line in the crossover region is seldom as unambiguous as it is in the idealized rate control system in the illustrative example. For example, an evaluation of a B-2 susceptibility to PIOs provides a realistic case showing that the Smith-Geddes criterion does not account for PIOs experienced by the B-2 unless the details of the slope computation are modified.[26]

Estimating the Frequency of Category I Oscillatory APC Events

The potential PIO frequency is very important for several reasons. First, it reflects the system characteristics that underlie the oscillation, and second, it points to changes that might be made to reduce the PIO tendency. It also indicates the most sensitive frequency regions of the closed-loop PVS, provides a basis for selecting test inputs, and is useful in several other ways. In all the cases and criteria treated here, PVS dynamics are extended-rigid-body characteristics and only the lower-frequency effects of higher-frequency modes are considered. In these situations, PIO frequency is always less than 1 Hz (3.14 rad/sec) when the pilot is operating in a compensatory manner, and it may be as high as, perhaps, 2.5 Hz (8 rad/sec) for fully-developed synchronous operations.

Alternative methods for estimating the frequency of Category I PIOs abound. The Smith-Geddes formula (Equation 6-3) comes close when the high frequency time lags are small. When time lags are larger, the estimate of PIO

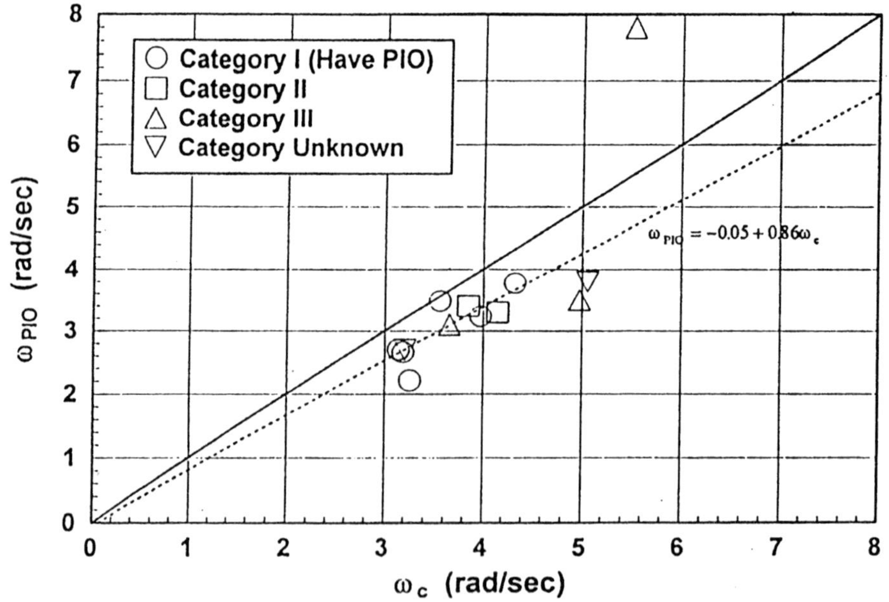

FIGURE 6-6 Correlation between Smith-Geddes criterion frequency and Have PIO flight data. Source: Klyde.[39]

frequency using the Smith-Geddes estimate for ω_c can be improved by using Equation 6-7. This approach is suggested not only by its successful fit to the Have PIO data but also by the (possible) coincidence that it is not too far off for the other aircraft represented in Figure 6-6. Because Equation 6-7 is purely empirical, it could, perhaps, be refined using additional PIO data.

A better way to make estimates when the pilot is operating in a compensatory mode is to apply the pilot-modeling routines to find the neutral stability frequency from specific pilot-model estimates for particular effective aircraft dynamics.[45] Although this method is more complicated than using Equation 6-3, it is straightforward and can also provide a good deal of information about pilot dynamic behavior, including pilot-adopted compensation, second-order effects of inceptors, and pseudo ratings and commentaries. In fact, this approach has so much to offer in terms of detailed understanding that the committee believes it should always be used in situations that exceed a threshold of concern. The potential accuracy of this procedure can be appreciated by using Bjorkman's estimates (based on a version of the general compensatory-pilot model) of the attitude-control resonant frequency (ω_r) for the Have PIO data.[5] The linear regression[42] relating these estimates to the (later) observed PIO frequency data is:

$$\omega_{PIO} = 0.02 + 1.01\,\omega_r,\ r = 0.97 \qquad \text{(Equation 6-8)}$$

The correlation between ω_r and ω_{PIO} is excellent, as is the correlation coefficient, r for this restrictive data set. It also suggest that the Have PIO Category I PIOs were fundamentally compensatory in nature.

The quickest and least-complicated procedure for estimating ω_{PIO} using a pilot model that accounts for high frequency lags is to apply the crossover model to the Have PIO data with the result:

$$\omega_{PIO} = 0.33 + 0.97\,\omega_{ucm},\ r = 0.94 \qquad \text{(Equation 6-9)}$$

where ω_{ucm} is the neutral stability frequency [$\angle Y_p Y_c(j\omega_{ucm}) = -180$ degrees] as predicted by the crossover model. Thus, the elementary crossover model, combined with a rough first approximation of the effective time lag of the PVS, appears to capture enough of the underlying phenomena to provide a reasonable estimate of PIO frequency.

Another easy way to make an estimate of PIO frequency is to connect ω_{PIO} with the neutral stability frequency for the synchronous-pilot pitch-attitude control system. This is, of course, the ω_{180} frequency in the aircraft-bandwidth/phase delay definitions. McRuer[42] gives this relationship for the severe PIO data as

$$\omega_{PIO} = 0.13 + 1.11\,\omega_{180},\ r = 0.97 \qquad \text{(Equation 6-10)}$$

Thus, if this empirical equation can be generalized, the estimated PIO frequency is somewhat greater than 111 percent of the frequency predicted for a synchronous pilot interacting with the aircraft's attitude dynamics.

This result has some interesting implications. For example, the pilot, if operating primarily on attitude cues, must be providing a phase advance at the PIO frequency that more than offsets all of the internal time lags. An alternative explanation could be that the dominant cues available to the pilot in the Have PIO flights include pitch rate or another aircraft output variable (e.g., sight line) that leads attitude oscillations, thereby compensating for pilot time lags. The Bjorkman data are insufficient to decide among such speculations, although some time traces from other PIO sources indicate that pilot switching on rate cues may occur in some cases.[9,23]

For the present, one can interpret equations 6-7 and 6-10, respectively, as statements that the Smith-Geddes ω_c estimate is higher than the actual PIO frequency and that the ω_{180} neutral stability frequency for pure gain attitude control is lower than the actual PIO frequency. If these correlation's are shown to be generally correct, they could be useful, easily calculated bounds on Category I PIO frequencies. A useful rule of thumb might be to sum and average equations 6-7 and 6-10:

$$\omega_{PIO} = 0.04 + 0.55\,\omega_{180} + 0.43\,\omega_c \qquad \text{(Equation 6-11)}$$

Equation 6-11 implies that an estimate for Category I ω_{PIO} is not far from the mean of ω_{180} and the Smith-Geddes ω_c. When using this experimental relation, the investigator should remember the ancient principle of caveat emptor.

Neal-Smith Criteria and Modifications

The Neal-Smith approach is solidly based on closed-loop operations. However, the normal Neal-Smith boundaries are connected with flying qualities levels rather than PIO potential per se. In this context, PIO-potential is one factor but not the factor that leads to a non-Level 1 aircraft. Thus, Neal-Smith, as presently constituted, is not selective for PIO. However, suitable modifications to the boundaries might enable a Neal-Smith approach be used a criterion for PIO susceptibility.

Some work on modifying Neal-Smith Criteria has already been done by the Moscow Aviation Institute.[18] The Neal-Smith[53] and LAHOS[63] configurations were examined in piloted-simulator studies with tracking tasks, taking detailed measurements of pilot and pilot-vehicle dynamic characteristics as well as pilot CH PR and PIO rating. Neal-Smith-like boundaries were then developed using actual experimental data for the pilot lead (as a workload indicator) and a closed-loop PVS peak magnification ratio. Different boundaries were drawn for flying qualities levels and for PIOs. The PIO boundaries are shown in Figure 6-7.

Illustrative Example.

The Neal-Smith approach requires the analyst to estimate the open-loop pilot lead (or time lag) and the closed-loop system resonance using a particular pilot model. The rules for adjusting the pilot characteristics within the fixed-form model include constraints on the closed-loop system bandwidth and droop.[53] These rules have been applied to the idealized rate-command aircraft for a succession of effective time delays (τ_e). As summarized in Figure 6-8, as the delay increases there is a demand for more pilot lead and an increase in closed-loop resonance. This trend shows how the pilot might cope with increasing controlled-element time lags to maintain control precision (as defined by the closed-loop bandwidth) at a desired level. This example also shows how the Moscow Aviation Institute PIO boundaries can be used in the context of the trend line. The intersection of the boundary and the trend line occurs at an effective time delay of approximately 0.29 sec. This corresponds to a phase delay of 0.145 sec or an average phase rate of 104 degrees/Hz. The remarkably close agreement with the previous illustrative examples gives credence to the view that Neal-Smith concepts can be expanded to examine PIO-susceptibility trends.

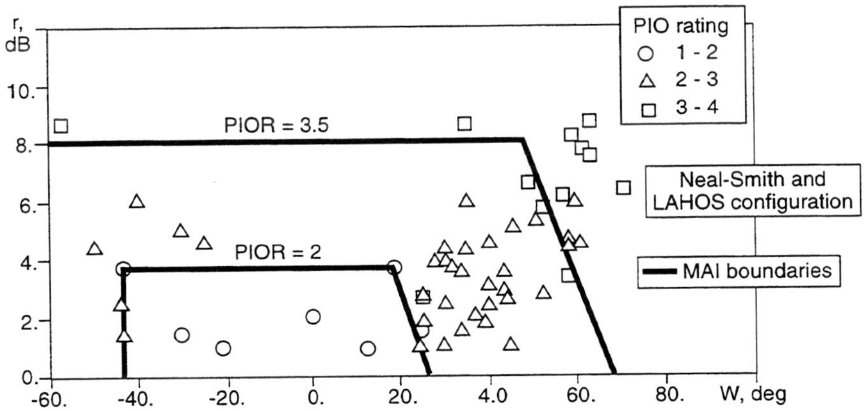

FIGURE 6-7 Moscow Aviation Institute PIO boundaries. Source: Efremov.[18]

Dropback

The Dropback parameter, $\Delta\theta_{peak}$, which is illustrated in Figure 6-9, deals with metrics, such as q_{peak}/q_{ss}, derived from the attitude response to step inputs. Dropback may not appear to be an accurate measure of closed-loop PVS response because, strictly speaking, it is an open-loop aircraft response. However, the Dropback characteristics $\Delta\theta_{peak}$ and q_{peak}/q_{ss} for K_c/s vehicle dynamics are zero. Then, when the effective vehicle dynamics (Y_c) become more complex and depart from a K_c /s-like character, they become larger. Dropback can thus be interpreted as a time-domain indicator of the degree of "K/s-ness" exhibited by a particular set of effective aircraft attitude dynamics. One facet of PVS resistance to PIO is insensitivity to variations in pilot gain, in the case of the ideal rate-command controlled element, for example. To the extent that an ideal PIO-insensitive aircraft has dynamics approximating K/s over a suitably prescribed frequency regime, the Dropback parameter can be used a measure of this feature of PIO susceptibility.

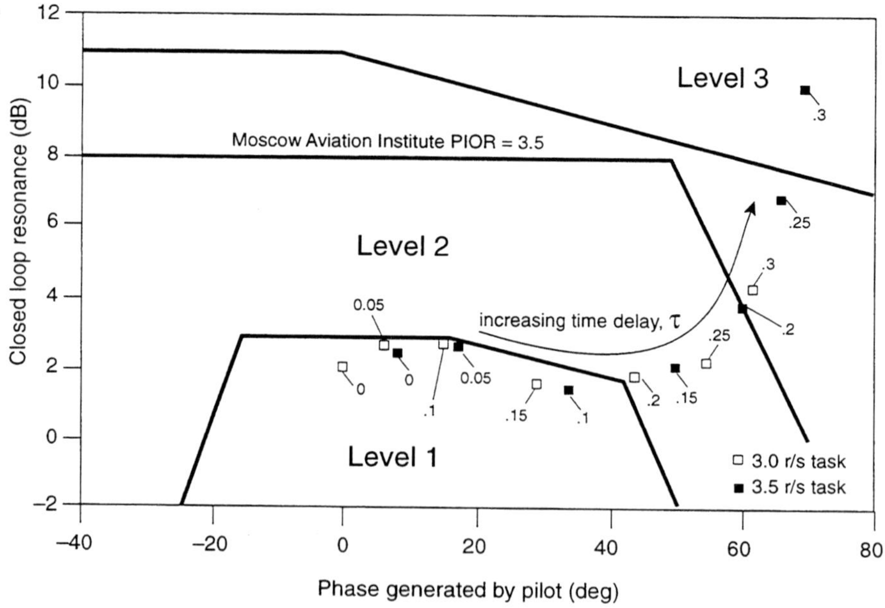

FIGURE 6-8 Neal-Smith trends with variation of effective delay for $K_c e^{-s\tau}/s$.

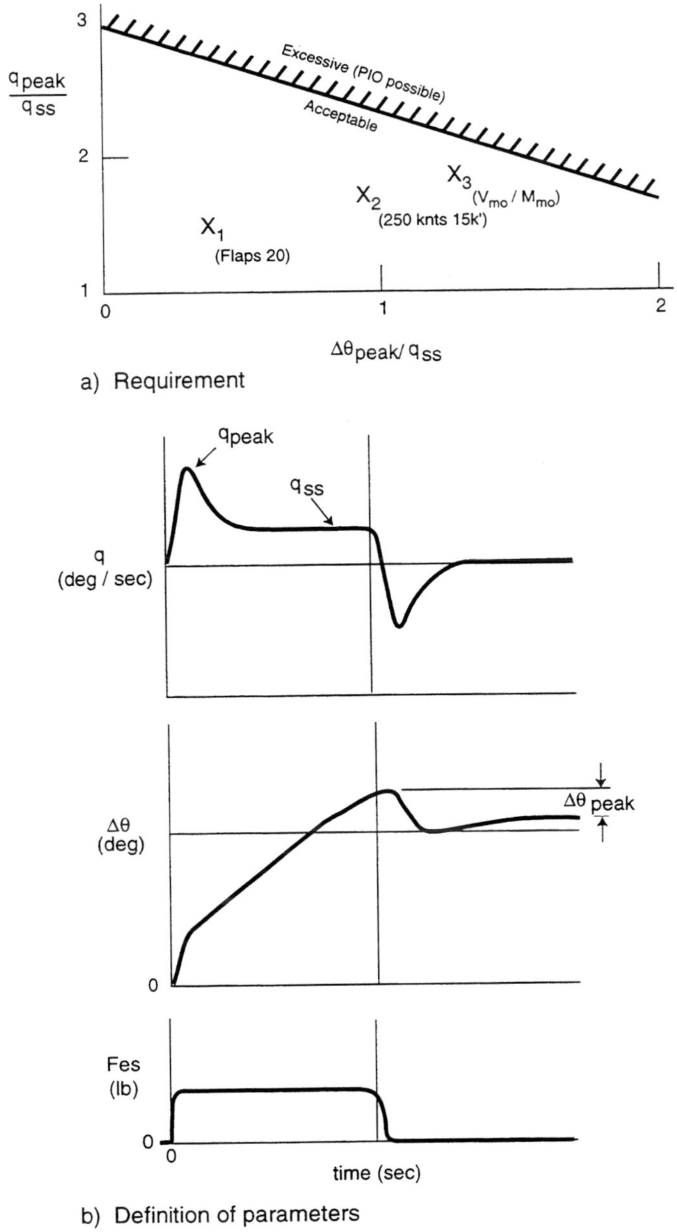

FIGURE 6-9 Pitch rate overshoot and pitch attitude dropback. Source: Nelson and Landes.[54]

Because the pulse applied as the test input is really two pulses separated by 10 sec, Dropback is not sensitive to high-frequency effective delays. For instance, the Dropback for the rate-command controlled element with an effective time delay of Equation 6-2 is zero, just as it is for a pure $Y_c = K_c/s$ rate command transfer function. The Dropback parameters, by themselves, are therefore insufficient as a PIO criterion. However, the combination of Dropback parameters and the average phase rate do provide a useful PIO criterion. As has already been noted in connection with Figures 6-2 and 6-3, Dropback can occasionally be used to justify eliminating otherwise awkward data.

The Dropback criterion boundary shown in Figure 6-9 was based primarily on data from fighter aircraft. The data points shown on the figure (x_1, x_2, x_3) are from flight tests of the Boeing 777 and correspond to the flight conditions added to Figure 6-3. They are shown here to justify the assertion that the Dropback parameter can also be applied fruitfully to FBW transport aircraft.

Because Dropback is a good measure of K/s character, it is applicable only to rate-type controlled elements; it will not apply directly to special controlled-element forms such as attitude command or flight-path command effective vehicle dynamics.

Extending Criteria to the Lateral Axis

The discussion so far has emphasized the dynamics of pilot control of the longitudinal axis. Some of the same metrics, criteria, and approaches have been examined for control of the lateral axis, although not to the same extent. Unfortunately, the research and detailed test and operational aircraft data bases for lateral-axis control are much more limited, and the effects of pilot-controller sensitivity are not as well accounted for. The most current and complete summary concludes that "PIO is unlikely if phase delay is less than 0.17 sec, as long as [controller] sensitivity is separately optimized; and PIO is likely always if phase delay is above about 0.17 sec."[48] A comparable value of average phase rate would be 122 degrees/Hz.

Mitchell and Hoh[48] also examined the Smith-Geddes criterion using the same experimental data on lateral-axis control. The Smith-Geddes criterion reliably predicted all but one of the PIO events. Unfortunately, a fair number of non-PIO susceptible systems were PIO-prone according to this criterion, once again indicating that the Smith-Geddes criterion may be overly conservative.

Two current reviews of assessment criteria have concluded that the lack of data on effective controlled element gain (i.e., cockpit-controller gain), especially for novel inceptors, is a major deficiency for assessing Category IPIOs.[39,48] Even the best set of optimum aircraft dynamics can become PIO-prone if the gain is too sensitive.[42] In past experiments, this variable has been fairly well controlled to be near optimum levels for conventional cockpit longitudinal-control devices. This has not been true of lateral control devices.

In the thorough flight investigations of PIO susceptibility conducted during the development phases of the Boeing 777 aircraft, Aircraft-Bandwidth/Phase Delay and Smith-Geddes Type III measures were examined for both the lateral and longitudinal control axes. A flight test series involving simulated refueling and other high-gain pilot experiments received a CH PR of 2 and a PIO rating of 1 to 2. The phase delay was always less than 0.14 sec when wheel position was used as the input. When the input was wheel force, the phase delay values increased markedly, from a minimum of 0.2 sec to 0.34 sec.

The bank-attitude-to-wheel-position phase angle, evaluated at the frequency specified by the Smith-Geddes criterion, did not fare as well as the phase delay. Although the data were clustered around −180 degrees, thereby indicating a marginal PIO tendency based on the Smith-Geddes criterion, the pilot evaluations during extensive simulation of refueling and other high-gain closed-loop tasks showed no PIO tendencies whatsoever.

Ongoing research to improve criteria has contributed to more comprehensive specifications by the military (see below) and the FAA. Even so, currently there are no specific requirements to conduct APC-related testing of either military or commercial aircraft during the development and certification process; specific procedures that address APC concerns are generally at the discretion of the manufacturer.

MILITARY STATUS AND TRENDS

Development of New Quantitative Requirements for MIL STD 1797

As initially issued, Military Flying Qualities Specification for Piloted Vehicle (MIL STD 1797) had qualitative PIO requirements that said, in effect, there shall be no PIOs resulting from the pilot's attempt to control the aircraft. There were also a significant number (16) of quantitative PIO-related requirements, although they were interspersed with other requirements that were not PIO-related. As a result, the PIO-related requirements did not stand out in any way.

In practice, the design goal for military aircraft is to meet Level 1 flying qualities requirements, but most aircraft demonstrate varying degrees of Level 2 flying qualities. There is no distinction among Level 1 flying qualities requirements in terms of importance. That is, each Level 1 requirement is presented as if it were of equal value to the mission objectives for the aircraft. The mission impact of the possible permutations and combinations of individual Level 1 and Level 2 flying qualities requirements is not known. Consequently, critical PIO-related requirements are "buried" among other, less important requirements. One purpose of the interim update of MIL STD 1797 was to add quantitative requirements that specifically address PIOs.[71] The update also emphasized requirements that are generally related to PIOs by calling them out again where PIO-specific requirements are presented. The quantitative Smith-Geddes requirement was added to the specification, although it only addresses linear PIO elements and is based on limited PIO data (essentially the Neal-Smith data base). These two changes are expected to result in proper attention being paid to factors that influence PIO tendencies.

Other efforts related to MIL STD 1797 include research into extending the linear PIO criteria to nonlinear PIO events. One approach is to seek a time-domain equivalent of the Neal-Smith frequency-domain criteria.[4] In this time-domain approach, nonlinear PIO events are addressed by placing restrictions directly on the time histories of relevant PVS inputs and outputs. Selection of an appropriate parameter for target acquisition time is used to define aggressiveness. Currently, aggressiveness is limited by its subjective nature. Further criteria development is being pursued by several major airframe developers. This work is expected to ensure that widest possible PIO experience and data base are considered for developing and validating newly proposed requirements.

Development of Verification Maneuver Requirements by the U.S. Air Force

It is unrealistic to assume that even comprehensive and well documented criteria can eliminate PIOs. Unknown triggers may create circumstances not previously covered by the criteria. Even so, good criteria can reduce the probability of encountering PIOs. This is particularly true when they are combined with reliable evaluation techniques that expose PIO tendencies early in the development process.

Unfortunately, current evaluation techniques are not adequate for either flight testing or simulations. The selection of a sufficiently demanding task that will inherently raise the pilot's gain and frequency response has been hindered by two real considerations: safety and "realistic" flying that doesn't provoke overwhelming criticism from pilots and others outside the flying qualities community. To gain acceptance of "unrealistic" tasks as necessary for evaluating PIO tendencies, the relationship and validity of the task in question to the PIO issue must be clearly established. To this end, flight test evaluation maneuvers are being developed.

Some tasks, including HQDT (handling qualities during tracking) and capture tasks, have already been added to the updated MIL STD 1797. The new flight-test evaluation maneuvers include HQDT tasks for the following mission tasks: air-to-air tracking, power approach, air-to-ground tracking, boom tracking, and formation flying. Clearly, HQDT and similar tasks, along with capture tasks, expose some PIO tendencies and can readily be extended to mission tasks other than air-to-air or air-to-ground tracking. An extensive discussion of the mission tasks and the HQDT version of these tasks is presented in Appendix A of the updated specification.[71] Properly performed, these tasks will increase the likelihood of discovering PIO tendencies in a safe and controlled fashion.

Test maneuvers should be challenging enough to force pilot gain to maximum levels while ensuring that flight safety is maintained. This dilemma is more significant for tasks requiring large control inputs, for recovery from extreme gust upsets, or for rate limiting cases, for example. Some PIO evaluations may only be possible with ground-based or in-flight simulation tests. However, additional work will be required to determine which modifications, if any, are necessary to validate that simulated tasks are reliable indicators of PIO tendencies. Research has been initiated to address these issues.

CRITERIA FOR ASSESSING OTHER CONDITIONS

Pilot-Aircraft Systems with Higher-Frequency Modes

The current status of APC criteria, as described in this chapter, is essentially satisfactory for assessing Category I PIO tendencies for a large class of effective aircraft dynamics. However, oscillations associated with higher-frequency modes are not covered. As Table 1-1 shows, such oscillations have occurred. Some were relatively mild, but others were severe and resulted in extreme situations involving structural failures. The latter have already required the addition of effective low-pass filtering (e.g., CH-53) or notch filtering (e.g., 777) to the PVS.

An experimental data base and appropriate pilot models can be used to estimate closed-loop characteristics for a PVS that includes flexible modes. Klyde, et al.,[39] have summarized pilot-centered phenomena (e.g., closed-loop control, vibration feedthrough, and remnant excitation), appropriate references to experimental data, and examples of analysis for the YF-12 and a large helicopter. The techniques and data provided there can be used to examine the need for remedial measures and to assess their utility.

The frequency range over which a pilot may have a significant effect extends to 3 Hz for direct, closed-loop control and to nearly 10 Hz for vibration feedthrough and remnant excitation effects.

Non-Oscillatory APC Events

The specter of novel, non-oscillatory APC events associated with new FCS features and functions made possible by FBW technology was raised in Chapter 2. These events tend to occur in situations near control limits that create discrepancies between what the aircraft is doing and the pilot's expectations. Several features associated with non-oscillatory APC events can be noted. The first focuses on the sharing of control effectors among control axes at or near the limits of authority of the control functions. The historical antecedents for shared control include longitudinal and lateral control on elevon, ailevator, and taileron control surfaces. On some modern, high-performance aircraft, shared control is further complicated by the addition of multifunction canards, flaps, thrust vectoring, etc. Although composite control effectors are not, in principle, a consequence of FBW control technology, they are made feasible in practice by FBW technology.

The second factor associated with non-oscillatory APC events is also enabled by FBW technology. This factor is the addition of novel functions, such as gust alleviation and maneuver load control, assorted limiting features (angle of attack, speed, load factor, etc.), and operating point (accelerating trim) control. At the limits of the operational envelopes for these functions, they can modify the pilot's direct authority over the control effectors as well as give rise to transient changes in the effective aircraft dynamics.

Finally, by its very nature, a FBW FCS separates the pilot from direct mechanical connections with the effectors. Situations, such as hitting rate limits while in tight closed-loop tracking tasks, can suddenly introduce a phase lag leading to a Category II PIO event (see Chapter 2 and Appendix C). In general, the control surface position can be far behind the pilot's command without the pilot's knowledge. Upon reversal of the pilot command, the surface may even continue in the opposite direction until the surface actuation system error is reduced to zero, at which point the surface will reverse direction. For large, sharply applied, open-loop pilot commands, this control divergence can produce an effective time delay of several hundred milliseconds, as exemplified by the JAS-39 accidents.

These features combine to make PVS behavior at the margins of the control-effector/control-function envelope a multidimensional surface of bewildering complexity. In most cases in which there are large effective time delays, the pilot's perceptions will undergo two successive steps. The first is, "Nothing I do matters; I'm disconnected from the control surfaces." This is followed by a period in which the pilot attempts to sort everything out and come up with a response. Because this time can be governed by multichoice reaction time, it can last for seconds rather than milliseconds. In the second JAS-39 accident, for example, the pilot left the airplane 5.9 seconds after the start of the PIO, when the time delay had reached 0.8 sec. This shows that on an initial APC encounter, the second step in pilot perception does not come easily. This phenomenon may underlie some of the three-dimensional PIOs described in Chapter 1. Resulting incidents and accidents will probably be ascribed to the "pilot overdriving the system."

Because there are many design choices and tradeoffs, there would appear to be no general, quantitative way to treat or assess non-oscillatory APC events that may be associated with non-harmonious limit envelopes. But design approaches can be adopted to ameliorate the situation. Thus, at one extreme, one can choose to reestablish a direct connection with the actuation system by requiring the FBW system to emulate a mechanical system. At another extreme, system logic can modify the authorities of various automatic functions as a function of the pilot's commands and the proximity to the limits, etc.

The important message here is that extremely limiting conditions on the effector and function envelope are inevitable and must be recognized and addressed, starting with a systematic and thorough examination of the myriad possible conditions that could exist near the limits of effector envelopes. Once potentially critical situations are recognized, design modifications, simulator assessments, and other methods of detecting and eliminating problematic conditions can follow.

Category II Assessments and Criteria

The conditions attending possible Category II PIOs caused by rate limiting can be identified using existing analytical and computational routines,[14,15,16,17,31,39,42,62] which can provide information about the frequency, amplitude, circumstances of onset, and other characteristics of PIOs of this type.

There were two primary reasons for establishing Category II as a separate category in which nonlinear rate limiting and/or position limiting are central factors in PIOs. First, a large number of PIOs have involved rate or position limiting. Second, a relatively simple, analysis-oriented approach can lead to the discovery of PIO potential in rate limiting or position limiting situations. The more general Category III includes events associated with more complex nonlinear phenomena (other than rate and position limiting) as well as transitions in effective aircraft dynamics.

Recent attention to rate limiting PIO situations makes the analysis procedures routine. The prevalence of rate limiting as a factor in severe PIOs in flight would seem to indicate that a preliminary search for Category II possibilities is a reasonable step in checking new designs. This search can be carried out at several levels of detail, including bench tests with actual software and hardware.

Pass/fail assessment criteria for new designs are not as well developed as analytic methods intended to discover possibilities, but a promising start has been made.[15,16,17] The approach used in these studies is to define a forbidden region in the gain/phase domain. The boundaries for this region are based primarily on an examination of a large number of configurations that exhibited Category II PIOs when the onset frequency appeared within those boundaries (Figure 6-10). The rate-limiting onset frequencies and the linear system characteristics are then used together to locate the possible onset of rate limiting on the gain/phase plot. Locations inside the forbidden region are PIO-prone. The concept is fundamentally sound, but the details currently depend on certain assumptions about the details of the PVS. Pilot-vehicle simulation studies to validate these assumptions have not yet been done.

CONCLUSIONS

In addition to the major findings and recommendations listed in Chapter 7, the committee generated a number of conclusions regarding APC design assessment criteria. The available Category I criteria contain a mix of complementary elements that can be used to highlight the importance of APC issues at many levels within design, development, and test organizations. In the current environment of substantial computational resources, it is reasonable and prudent to use all available criteria through the analysis phases of design. During subsequent design, development, and test phases, partial assessments can be made using the most convenient tools for the task at hand, interpreted in

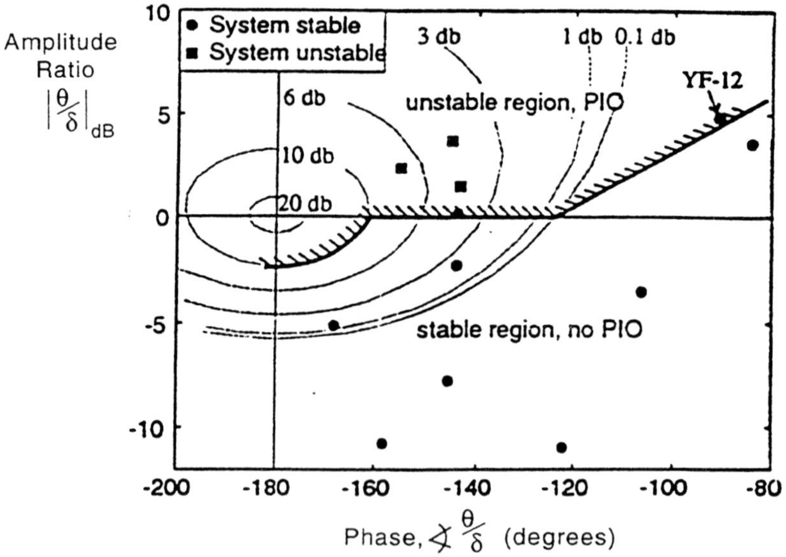

FIGURE 6-10 Tentative forbidden zones for Category II PIOs. Source: Duda.[15]

the context of the more complete data set available from the analysis phases. For example, dropback as a time-domain measure might be more convenient for assessing flight test tasks than the more elaborate frequency sweeps required for Aircraft-Bandwidth/Phase Delay or other frequency-domain measures.

Some of the F-16 and YF-22 control system parameters have not correlated well with some available criteria. Yet the YF-22 test pilots were very pleased with the aircraft's handling qualities. This anomalous history should be taken into account when criteria are chosen and the control system structure is selected. Even so, the structure of the F-22 control system has been redesigned to better correlate with handling qualities and APC criteria.

It would be prudent for designers to consider more elaborate analyses, simulations, and tests if most initial approaches show even marginal APC potential. Designers should also recognize that all available criteria assume that the effective controlled element gain is optimized. In addition, designers should remain sensitive to the risk posed by Category II and III APC events, even if available criteria indicate satisfactory performance with respect to Category I APC events. For example, design assessments should search for situations that may encourage non-oscillatory APC events caused by a lack of harmony between pilot expectations and control system actions, especially in situations that are on or near the margins of control-effector/control-function envelopes.

The Aircraft-Bandwidth/Phase Delay and ω_{180}/Average Phase Rate criteria can be determined unambiguously only if flexible modes and/or quadratic dipole pairs appear only at frequencies well above $2\omega_{180}$. A shortcoming with the Smith-Geddes Attitude-Dominant Type III criterion in its current formulation is that, on occasion, an artistic interpretation must be made to determine the amplitude-ratio slope (m).

The Smith-Geddes Type III criterion tends to be over conservative, sometimes warning of PIO susceptibility when experience has shown it to be unlikely. However, an aircraft that clears the Aircraft-Bandwidth/Phase Delay, Smith-Geddes Type III, and Gain/Phase Template criteria will have minimal risk of experiencing Category I APC events.

Two combinations of criteria are particularly useful for conducting pass/fail assessments of susceptibility to Category I APC events: (1) Dropback plus Aircraft-Bandwidth/Phase Delay criteria, and (2) Dropback plus Gain/Phase Template, including ω_{180}/Average Phase Rate. These combinations can help designers to distinguish which aircraft are prone to Category I APC events. They are also directly useful for designing aircraft to avoid APC.

It is relatively easy to estimate the frequency region for Category I PIOs. The Smith-Geddes Type III criterion seems to provide a useful upper bound on PIO frequency. The synchronous-pilot frequency (i.e., the –180 degree phase frequency for the effective aircraft dynamics) may provide a lower bound.

There are several areas where available criteria need to be improved. For example, the Smith-Geddes Type III frequency formulation should be fine tuned to take more current data into account. This would make the Smith-Geddes Type III criteria less restrictive and thus a better discriminator on a pass/fail basis. Similarly, Aircraft-Bandwidth/Phase Delay boundaries should continue to be reviewed and adjusted to accommodate new data. Also, because of the unique insights offered by the Neal-Smith criteria, the recent promising modifications to them should be extended and exploited.

The utility of available criteria could also be improved by more fully exploring the effects of angular and linear accelerations, as well as other non-attitude-sensitive cues, on sensitivity and susceptibility to Category I APC events. There is some evidence that these cues have a second-order, yet beneficial, impact. If this is true, the existing attitude-dominant measures and criteria may suffice only as conservative criteria. Normal acceleration at the pilot's location has long been considered to be an important or even central cue in closed-loop oscillatory behavior. Indeed, the Smith-Geddes Type I theory (which this report does not address) offers an elementary criterion for assessing acceleration feedback effects on PIO susceptibility that should be checked for completeness.[66]

Additional research is especially important on design assessment criteria for Category II and III PIOs and non-oscillatory APC events. This research should include experiments and the development of new analysis methods. Promising Category II assessment criteria, in particular, should be subjected to experimental verification.

7

Findings and Recommendations

The findings and recommendations of the Committee on the Effects of Aircraft-Pilot Coupling on Flight Safety were developed during deliberations that included consideration of all information collected by the committee. The findings and recommendations reflect current levels of understanding about APC and the processes currently used to mitigate the risks posed by adverse APC events. Implementation of the recommendations would improve aviation safety now and in the future by improving the effectiveness of APC-related design and test procedures, specifications, certification standards, training, and research. The rationale for each of the committee's findings and recommendations appears in the chapter indicated by the chapter heading.

CHAPTER 1
AIRCRAFT-PILOT COUPLING PROBLEMS: DEFINITIONS, DESCRIPTIONS, AND HISTORY

Finding 1-1. Adverse APC events are rare, unintended, and unexpected oscillations or divergences of the pilot-aircraft system. Adverse APC events are fundamentally interactive and occur during highly demanding tasks when environmental, pilot, or aircraft dynamic changes create or trigger mismatches between actual and expected aircraft responses.

Finding 1-2. APC problems are often associated with the introduction of new designs, technologies, functions, or complexities. APC problems can also arise when existing aircraft are tasked with new operational missions for which APC susceptibility has not been assessed during development testing. (This can occur when commercial aircraft are converted to military use.) New technologies, such as FBW and fly-by-light FCSs, are constantly being incorporated into aircraft. As a result, opportunities for APC are likely to persist or even increase, and greater vigilance is necessary to ensure that new technologies do not inadvertently increase the susceptibility of new aircraft to APC events.

Finding 1-3. APC problems have occurred more often in military and experimental aircraft, which have traditionally introduced advanced technologies, than in civil aircraft.

Finding 1-4. Recently, civil and military transport FBW aircraft have experienced APC problems during development and testing, and some APC events have occurred in recent commercial aircraft service, although they may not always have been recognized as such.

Finding 1-5. A recent trend in APC is that events have been associated with the introduction of FBW and aircraft automation systems.

CHAPTER 2
VARIETIES OF AIRCRAFT-PILOT COUPLING EXPERIENCE

Finding 2-1. There are two major types of severe APC events—PIOs and non-oscillatory APC events.

Finding 2-2. From the pilot's perspective, there are three varieties of PIOs:

- relatively benign, initial or early encounters that occur when the pilot is learning to adapt to the effective aircraft dynamics
- severe, potentially dangerous oscillations stemming from a combination of extreme task demands, which require very high gain in the PVS, and deficiencies in the effective aircraft dynamics, such as excessive time lag
- severe, potentially dangerous oscillations occasioned by pilot commands that are usually motivated by task demands and are large enough to cause a major nonlinear change (flying qualities cliff) in the effective aircraft dynamics

Finding 2-3. Conflicting priorities between different control authorities acting on the same effector can cause a severe safety risk or flying qualities cliff when the system is operating at or near the limiting conditions of the effector's positions or rates, thereby creating a latent non-linearity in the effective aircraft dynamics for an unsuspecting pilot.

Finding 2-4. Non-oscillatory APC events are also likely to occur or to be triggered when the aircraft trim is inconsistent with the pilot's expectations.

Recommendation 2-1. An active and aggressive search for APC tendencies, as contrasted with an incremental approach, should be included in efforts to discover cliff-like APC tendencies.

Recommendation 2-2. Reliable test procedures should be developed to discover and explore in detail sudden shifts in the PVS.

CHAPTER 3
AIRCRAFT-PILOT COUPLING AS A CURRENT PROBLEM IN AVIATION

Finding 3-1. With current test data recording and instrumentation equipment, APC events discovered in flight testing have almost always been defined well enough to permit detailed analysis and the development of fixes for the specific cause or causes.

Finding 3-2. Operational aircraft are not usually equipped with flight data collection systems that can provide investigators with enough data to discern whether APC was a causal factor in an accident or incident.

Finding 3-3. New generation flight data recorders provide enough data to analyze flight events encountered by civil transport aircraft in great detail. However, the proposed sampling rates may be inadequate for determining APC triggering events.

Finding 3-4. APC accidents and incidents have occurred when the pilot suddenly and unexpectedly was required to take manual control, often when the autopilot was disengaged while the aircraft was in a grossly out-of-trim condition of which the pilot was unaware.

Finding 3-5. Operational line pilots have little or no exposure to APC potential and are not trained to recognize the initial symptoms or to understand that APC does not imply poor airmanship. This may limit reporting of APC events.

Recommendation 3-1. A system should be developed whereby pilots are enabled and encouraged to report unusual events, including events that result from their inadvertent actions, without fear of punitive action. In particular, renewed efforts should be made to improve reporting of APC events by pilots to existing safety reporting systems, such as the Aviation Safety Reporting System.

Recommendation 3-2. Airlines should analyze flight data recorders for adverse events to detect trends and head off incidents and accidents before they occur.

Recommendation 3-3. The parameters recorded by flight data recorders and the sampling rates used should be selected to enable identification of APC events and causes.

CHAPTER 4
PRECLUDING ADVERSE AIRCRAFT-PILOT COUPLING EVENTS

Finding 4-1. The approaches used to address APC risk are inconsistent throughout the civil and military aviation communities. The incidence of APC events could be reduced through more effective and consistent use of existing tools and capabilities during design, analysis, simulation, and testing.

Finding 4-2. Currently, the FAA has no structured criteria for assessing adverse APC events during the certification process.

Finding 4-3. Over the years, the results of a great many separate development efforts, exemplified in this study by the Boeing 777 and the F-14 backup flight control module (see Chapter 2), have independently arrived at the conclusion that testing with high-gain pilot tasks oriented toward discovering APC tendencies is necessary for adequately exploring the APC characteristics of modern aircraft.

Finding 4-4. There are no widely accepted analysis and test guidelines for APC tendencies. As a result, even when APC-related tests are authorized and funded, test procedures are sometimes based on the personal experiences and preferences of the test personnel. Current practices do not systematically integrate design-team efforts to address APC issues early on, nor do they consistently make the best use of early indications that a problem may exist.

Recommendation 4-1. Insufficient attention to APC phenomena generally seems to be associated with a lack of understanding and relevant experience.

This shortcoming should be addressed through improved education about APC phenomena for pilots and other personnel involved in aircraft design, simulation, testing, certification, operation, and accident investigation.

Recommendation 4-2. A disciplined and structured approach should be taken in the design, development, testing, and certification stages to maximize the effectiveness of existing techniques for mitigating the risk of adverse APC tendencies and for expediting the incorporation of new techniques as they become available. This is especially important in areas where effective procedures and standards do not currently exist (e.g., FAA certification standards).

Recommendation 4-3. Organizations should adopt and implement risk minimization techniques in design and development policies, processes, and procedures. These techniques should be tailored and routinely updated to accommodate applications of newly developed technologies.

Recommendation 4-4. Appropriate analysis and simulation should be conducted throughout all program phases. Highly demanding tasks with known and suspected triggering events should be included in simulation, flight test, and certification; this is critical to mitigating APC risk.

Recommendation 4-5. In the interest of aviation safety, the free exchange of APC-related information on design and manufacturing processes and on aircraft performance characteristics should be encouraged throughout the military and civil aviation communities, nationally and internationally.

CHAPTER 5
SIMULATION AND ANALYSIS OF THE PILOT-VEHICLE SYSTEM

Simulation

Finding 5-1. Non-real-time, fixed-base, moving-base, and in-flight simulation tools can all play effective, complementary roles in discovering and understanding APC tendencies, as well as aiding in the assessment and partial validation of possible solutions. During simulations, APC potential is often indicated by subtle factors, such as increased pilot workload or sensitivity of the PVS to changes in aggressiveness. Actual PIOs or non-oscillatory APC events may not be found in all piloted simulations.

Finding 5-2. Situations that appear to be susceptible to APC events have sometimes been ignored on the basis that "pilots will not (or do not) fly like that."

Finding 5-3. Pilots who have a range of experience and who have been sensitized to look for APC events are crucial to the effective use of piloted simulations and development testing. More than two or three pilots must be involved for a thorough examination of marginal conditions.

Finding 5-4. Incremental expansion of a task or function envelop may not be effective for discovering Category II and III PIOs and some other types of APC events.

Analysis

Finding 5-5. When state-of-the-art PIO analysis tools and procedures are properly used, they are helpful for making a first cut in the APC discovery process, uncovering conditions likely to produce APC events, guiding more detailed and focused piloted-simulations, and generalizing experimental results via interpolation and extrapolation.

Finding 5-6. The weakest points in pilot-vehicle analysis for APC situations are pilot models that describe transient conditions in PIO onsets associated with changes in the controlled element. Not enough fundamental experimental data are available to build adequate models for these transient phases.

Finding 5-7. Although analytical approaches are available to address Category III situations, they have not yet been validated experimentally.

Recommendations

Recommendation 5-1. Existing simulation and analysis tools, including their joint use as complementary procedures, should be refined to be more specific and selective. Validating simulation details, protocols, and tasks and collecting and correlating them with flight test results should be given high priority.

Recommendation 5-2. A high priority should also be assigned to collecting data that can be used to validate existing analytic tools and to provide the empirical bases for new ones.

Recommendation 5-3. Tasks should be selected not only to be representative of nominal flight conditions, but also to explore the boundaries and extreme situations that may lead to APC events. Situations that cause APC events should not be eliminated because "pilots will not (or do not) fly like that."

Recommendation 5-4. A "discovery search" stage that encourages exploratory behavior by the pilot in search of PIOs and non-oscillatory APC events should be part of piloted simulation. This should include carefree flying as well as deliberate attempts to induce and explore APC tendencies (e.g., control reversals at PIO frequencies).

CHAPTER 6
CRITERIA FOR ASSESSING AIRCRAFT-PILOT COUPLING POTENTIAL

Finding 6-1. The measures and metrics used in Aircraft-Bandwidth/Phase Delay, Gain/Phase Template and Average Phase Rate, and Smith-Geddes Attitude-Dominant Type III criteria offer relevant and valuable insights for assessing and understanding attitude-dominant Category I PIO potentials. The Dropback and modified Neal-Smith criteria can also play important supplementary roles. Thus, each has something to offer in providing insights, pinpointing troublesome areas, and enhancing understanding. However, none is sufficient to predict with absolute accuracy the presence or absence of Category I PIO potential in either the pitch or lateral axis.

Finding 6-2. There are no validated metrics or criteria applicable to Category II and III PIO phenomena or non-oscillatory APC events. Such criteria are critical to a full assessment of the APC potential of new commercial and military aircraft.

Recommendation 6-1. An eclectic approach that applies a mix of criteria should be used for design assessment.

Recommendation 6-2. The current boundaries used to predict Category I PIO tendencies should be fine tuned to reduce known shortcomings. Boundaries should be adjusted from time to time to accommodate new data.

Recommendation 6-3. Research to develop design assessment criteria and analysis tools should focus on Category II and III PIOs and non-oscillatory APC events. Additional research is also needed to extend the application of existing criteria to the lateral axis. This research should combine experiments with the development of effective mathematical analysis methods capable of rationalizing and emulating the experimental results.

Recommendation 6-4. Existing specification and certification standards for military and commercial aircraft should be updated periodically to reflect advances in APC assessment criteria and testing techniques.

APPENDICES

APPENDIX A

Biographical Sketches of Committee Members

Duane T. McRuer (chair) is concurrently an independent consultant and chairman of Systems Technology, Incorporated (STI). He received his undergraduate and graduate education at the California Institute of Technology. Since 1950, Mr. McRuer's research has been focused on aerospace and ground vehicle and human pilot dynamics, automatic and manual vehicular control, and vehicle flying/handling qualities. He has published more than 125 technical papers and seven books, including *Analysis of Nonlinear Control Systems* (Wiley, 1961; Dover, 1971) and *Aircraft Dynamics and Automatics Control* (Princeton, 1973). He has also been involved with applications of these topics in more than 50 aerospace and land vehicles, and he has five patents on flight control and stability augmentation systems. Besides a career as president and technical director of STI (until 1993), he has been a Regent's Lecturer at the University of California, Santa Barbara, and was the 1992–1993 Hunsaker Professor at the Massachusetts Institute of Technology (MIT).

Mr. McRuer's past service for various governmental and professional societies includes terms as president of the American Automatic Control Council and chairman of the National Research Council Aeronautics and Space Engineering Board, the American Institute of Aeronautics and Astronautics (AIAA) Technical Committee on Guidance and Control, and the Society of Automotive Engineers (SAE) Aerospace Control and Guidance Systems Committee. He is currently on the National Aeronautics and Space Administration (NASA) Advisory Council. He is a fellow of the AIAA, Institute of Electrical and Electronic Engineers (IEEE), SAE, and the Human Factors and Ergonomics Society and a member of the National Academy of Engineering. Other honors include the Caltech Distinguished Alumni Award, the NASA Distinguished Public Service Medal, the AIAA Mechanical Mechanics and Control of Flight Award, the Franklin Institute's Levy Medal, and the Human Factors and Ergonomics Society Alexander Williams Award.

Carl S. Droste is the director of the Systems Integration Center of the Product Engineering Department at Lockheed Martin Tactical Aircraft Systems in Fort Worth, Texas. The Systems Integration Center is responsible for integrating flight control systems, among other things. Dr. Droste has worked at Lockheed Martin for more than 29 years. For more than 15 years, he was manager of the Flight Control Systems Section. Section activities spanned the full range of flight control system development, including functional responsibility for the F-111, the F-16, the AFTI/F-16, the F-16XL, the A-12, and the YF-22 programs. Dr. Droste received his undergraduate degrees from Rice University and his graduate degrees from Texas A & M University. He is a member of the IEEE and the SAE, where he serves on the Aerospace Control and Guidance Systems Committee.

R. John Hansman is a professor in the Department of Aeronautics and Astronautics at MIT, where he is head of the Humans and Automation Division. He also directs the MIT Aeronautical Systems Laboratory and the MIT International Center for Air Transportation. He has been a member of the faculty since receiving an interdisciplinary Ph.D. in physics, meteorology, electrical engineering, and aeronautical engineering from MIT in 1982. Since 1980, Dr. Hansman's research has been focused on a broad range of flight safety topics, ranging from aviation weather hazards, such as icing and windshear, to instrumentation and pilot-vehicle interface issues. He is the author of more than 90 technical papers in these areas and holds five patents. He is the recipient of the AIAA Losey Atmospheric Sciences Award for his work on the mitigation of aviation weather hazards. He has also received the Presidential Young Investigator Award and the OSTIV (Organisation Scientifique et Technique Internationale du Vol a Voile) Diploma. Dr. Hansman has more than 4,600 hours of flight experience in airplanes, helicopters, and sailplanes. He is an associate editor of the Journal of Aircraft and the Air Traffic Control Quarterly.

Dr. Hansman is an associate fellow of the AIAA and a former director of the Soaring Society of America. He is also a member of the Human Factors Society, Phi Beta Kappa, Sigma Xi, and the American Physical Society. He has served on numerous advisory and technical committees, including the Congressional Aeronautical Advisory Committee, the AIAA Atmospheric Environment Technical Committee, and the Federal Aviation Administration Research and Development Subcommittee on the National Airspace System.

Ronald A. Hess is a professor in the Department of Mechanical and Aeronautical Engineering at the University of California, Davis (UCD). He has been a member of the UCD faculty since 1982. Prior to his current academic position, Dr. Hess was a research scientist at NASA Ames Research Center, where he conducted research in the flight control and handling qualities of vertical and short takeoff and landing aircraft and rotorcraft. He is an associate fellow of the AIAA, a senior member of the IEEE, and a member of the American Helicopter Society. Dr. Hess is an associate editor of the Journal of Aircraft and the IEEE Transactions on Systems, Man, and Cybernetics. He is also a registered professional engineer in the state of California.

David P. LeMaster is chief of the Flight Control Division, Flight Dynamics Directorate, Wright Laboratory, at Wright-Patterson Air Force Base, Ohio. In this position since January 1993, Mr. LeMaster has led Air Force flight control and pilot-vehicle interface technology development for fixed-wing military flight vehicles. From 1988 to 1993, he was chief, Flight Technology Division, Flight Systems Engineering Directorate, Aeronautical Systems Center, responsible for aerodynamic and flight control system development and acquisition for aeronautical weapons systems. Between 1984 and 1988, Mr. LeMaster was director of engineering, F-16 System Program Office, Aeronautical Systems Center. In this position, he was responsible for all engineering support for F-16 block 10 and 25 configurations in the operational fleet, development and production of the F-16 block 30 and 40 configurations, and advanced development planning for the F-16 block 50 configuration. Earlier in his career, Mr. LeMaster received a Master of Science degree in the management of technology from MIT.

Stuart Matthews is chairman, president, and chief executive officer of the Flight Safety Foundation, a long-established international nonprofit organization that acts as an independent industry think tank on aviation safety. Born in London, England, Mr. Matthews has more than 43 years of aviation industry experience. He spent 15 years in the British manufacturing industry as an advanced project design engineer and in other positions, including a period working on the Concorde program. This was followed by seven years with British Caledonian Airways, where he was responsible for corporate and fleet planning. In 1974, he was invited by Fokker Aircraft in the Netherlands to establish a U.S. subsidiary company based in Washington, D.C. As president of Fokker USA, for the next 20 years Mr. Matthews looked after all of the company's business and marketing activities in North America, placing some 300 aircraft in the process. He was elected chairman of the Flight Safety Foundation in 1989 and, when he retired from Fokker in 1994, he was also appointed president and chief executive officer. Mr. Matthews is a chartered engineer, a fellow of the Royal Aeronautical Society, a fellow of the Chartered Institute of Transport, and an associate fellow of the AIAA. Upon his retirement from Fokker, he was knighted by the Queen of the Netherlands for his services to aviation.

John D. (Jack) McDonnell is director of vehicle management systems at McDonnell Douglas Corporation. He has been with McDonnell Douglas for 28 years, working on the design, development, testing, and certification of the DC-10 and MD-80 and managing the research and development of advanced flight control systems, avionics, and cockpit designs. Previously, Mr. McDonnell spent 10 years at STI working on analytical pilot models, pilot rating scales, and a variety of flight-control-related systems, such as approach power compensators, and Fresnel landing system stabilization strategies. He has B.S. and M.S. degrees in engineering from the University of California–Los Angeles. He is a member of Tau Beta Pi, the SAE Aerospace Control and Guidance Systems Committee, and NASA's Aeronautics Research and Technology Subcommittee on Guidance and Control.

James McWha is chief engineer of flight systems at Boeing Commercial Airplane Group, where he is responsible for all flight deck and flight controls activities. He has been with Boeing for 30 years, having worked on each of the current production airplanes. He was chief engineer for flight controls throughout development of the 777, Boeing's first fully fly-by-wire commercial airplane. Prior to Boeing, Mr. McWha worked for Short Brothers in Northern Ireland for four years after graduation from Queen's University, Belfast. Mr. McWha is a member of the AIAA, vice chairman of one of the SAE control and guidance subcommittees, and a member of the Flight Controls and Guidance Panel of NASA's Aeronautics Research and Technology Subcommittee.

William W. Melvin has a B.S. degree in mechanical engineering from the University of Texas. He was a patrol plane commander and transport plane commander in the U.S. Navy and retired from Delta Air Lines as a captain after 33 years of service. He was active in air safety with the Air Line Pilots Association (ALPA), serving as chairman of the Airworthiness and Performance Committee. He is the author and co-author of numerous articles and technical papers on aircraft performance. He has served on many industry committees, including the National Research Council Committee on Wind Shear in 1982, and has been a consultant to the Aero-Astronautics Group of Rice University and the National Institute of Standards Technology. Mr. Melvin is the recipient of a Flight Safety Foundation Award (1976), ALPA Annual Air Safety Award (1977), ALPA Air Safety Outstanding Service Award (1981), International Federation of Air Line Pilots Associations

(IFALPA) Scroll of Merit (1986), Aviation Week and Space Technology/Flight Safety Foundation Award (1993) and IFALPA Clarence N. Sayen Award (1994). He is co-recipient, with Dr. Angelo Miele and Dr. Tong Wang, of the O. Hugo Schuck award from the American Controls Conference (1989) for the best paper of 1988.

Richard W. Pew is principal scientist and manager of the Cognitive Sciences and Systems Department at BBN Corporation in Cambridge Massachusetts. Dr. Pew has 35 years of experience in human factors, human performance, and experimental psychology as they relate to systems design and development. He spent 11 years on the faculty of the Psychology Department at the University of Michigan where he was involved in teaching, research, and consulting before he moved to BBN in 1974. Throughout his career, Dr. Pew has been involved in the development and utilization of human performance models and in the conduct of experimental and field studies of human performance in applied settings. Dr. Pew was the first chairman of the National Research Council Committee on Human Factors. He has also been president of the Human Factors Society, chairman of the Biosciences Panel of the Air Force Scientific Advisory Board, and president of Division 21 of the American Psychological Association, the division concerned with engineering psychology.

APPENDIX B

Participants in Committee Meetings

In addition to committee members, liaisons, and staff (see page iii), the following individuals participated in meetings held by the Committee on the Effects of Aircraft-Pilot Coupling on Flight Safety. Presentation topics are also listed for outside speakers.

Main Workshop
November 27–29, 1995

Speakers

Avoiding Triggers: Pilot Expectations and Human Performance Considerations
Kathy Abbott, Langley Research Center
Key Factors to Cover in Flight- and Ground-Based Simulations
Randall Bailey and Michael Parrag, Calspan Corporation
Simulator Use to Minimize/Eliminate APC Tendencies; Test Pilot Preparation to Test for Aircraft Pilot Coupling
Jon Beesley, Lockheed Martin Tactical Aircraft Systems
Commercial Airline Operating Experience
Brent Blackwell, American Airlines
Commercial Airline Operating Experience
John Brown, Northwest Airlines
Experience with Ground- and Flight-Based Simulations of APC
Dwain Deets, Dryden Flight Research Center

YF-22 Experience and the F-22 APC Design Process
Jeffrey Harris, Lockheed Martin Tactical Aircraft Systems
Quantifying the Pilot's Contribution to Flight Safety
John Hodgkinson, McDonnell Douglas
Potential High Altitude Handling Qualities Criteria for Transport Aircraft
Roger Hoh, Hoh Aeronautics
C-17 Flying Qualities and APC Experience during the Development Process
Eric Kendall, McDonnell Douglas Transport Aircraft Research Center
Unified PIO (Pilot-Induced Oscillation) Programs; MIL STD 1797A
Dave Leggett, Wright Laboratory
Comparative Evaluation of Predicted Flying Qualities Boundaries Using Ground and Airborne Simulators
Tom Melody, Douglas Aircraft Company
APC Criteria and Prediction Techniques
Dave Mitchell and Roger Hoh, Hoh Aeronautics
YF-22 Mishap and Discussion of Other PIOs
Dave Moorhouse, Wright Laboratory
Boeing 777 Development and APC Assessment
Tim Nelson, Boeing Commercial Airplane Group
Design, Development, and Certification of the MD-11
Jeff Preston, McDonnell Douglas Aerospace
NTSB Experience with APC in Civil Aircraft Accidents and Incidents
Jim Ritter, National Transportation Safety Board
Critique of the Process
Ralph Smith, High Plains Engineering
Ground and Flight Simulation Capabilities
Rogers Smith, Dryden Flight Research Center

Other Participants

Donald Armstrong, FAA/Los Angeles Aircraft Certification
Irving Ashkenas, National Academy of Engineering
Dan Bower, National Transportation Safety Board
John Clark, National Transportation Safety Board
George Cooper, National Academy of Engineering
J. L. Denning, U.K. Civil Aviation Authority
H. J. Hickey, Jr., U.S Air Force Aeronautical Systems Center
Tom Imrich, Federal Aviation Administration
Jim Ritter, National Transportation Safety Board
Melvin Rogers, Federal Aviation Administration
Tom Melody, Douglas Aircraft Company
Wayne Thor, Wright Laboratory

Secondary Workshop
March 21–22, 1996

Speakers

Recent and Future Aircraft-Pilot Coupling Research at Deutsche Forschungsanstalt für Luft-und Raumfahrt e.V. (DLR) (Collected Material)
Peter Hamel, DLR
Probing APC Susceptibility through HQDT
LCDR Robert Niewoehner, F-18 E/F Integrated Test Team, U.S. Navy
Unified PIO Program Status Review
Wayne Thor, Wright Laboratory

Other Participants

Guy Thiel, Federal Aviation Administration, Los Angeles Aircraft Certification Office

Southern California Fact-Finding Trip
March 18–19, 1996

The committee chairman and NASA technical liaison met with the following individuals during a fact-finding trip to Dryden Fight Research Center, Air Force Flight Test Center, and the National Test Pilot School.

Meeting at Dryden Flight Research Center

Kathy Bahn, Dryden Flight Research Center
John Bosworth, Dryden Flight Research Center
Robert Clarke, Dryden Flight Research Center
Keith Hoffler, Dryden Flight Research Center
Joe Pahle, Dryden Flight Research Center
Patrick Stoliker, Dryden Flight Research Center
Keith Weichman, Dryden Flight Research Center

Meeting at the Air Force Flight Test Center

Yvonne Des Lauriers, Air Force Flight Test Center
Kirk Harwood, Air Force Flight Test Center

Brian Hobbs, Air Force Flight Test Center
Robert Lee, Air Force Flight Test Center
John Manke, Air Force Flight Test Center
Lee Peron, Air Force Flight Test Center
Paul Sorokowski, Air Force Flight Test Center
Tom Speer, Air Force Flight Test Center
Fred Webster, Air Force Flight Test Center
Kathy Wood, Air Force Flight Test Center

Meeting at the National Test Pilot School

Ralph Smith, High Plains Engineering
Sean Roberts, National Test Pilot School

European Fact-Finding Trip
April 27–May 7, 1996

The committee chairman and NASA technical liaison met with the following individuals during a fact-finding trip to Europe.

Meeting at Aerospatiale, Toulouse Plant

Dominique Chatrenet, Aerospatiale
Pierre Fabre, Aerospatiale
Christian Favre, Aerospatiale
Jacques Rosay, Airbus Industrie

Meeting at British Aerospace Defence, Military Aircraft Division

Keith McKay, British Aerospace Defence
Chris Fielding, British Aerospace Defence
Andy Holden, British Aerospace Defence
Neil Smith, British Aerospace Defence
Terry D. Smith, British Aerospace Defence
Mike J. Walker, British Aerospace Defence
John Gibson, British Aerospace Defence (retired)

Meeting at U.K. Department of Transport, Air Accidents Investigation Branch

Ken Smart, Air Accidents Investigation Branch
David F. King, Air Accidents Investigation Branch
Dick Vance, Air Accidents Investigation Branch
Jim Passmore, British Airways

Meeting at Saab Military Aircraft

Erik Kullberg, Saab Military Aircraft
Per-Olov Elgcrona, Saab Military Aircraft
John Enhagen, Saab Military Aircraft
Kenneth Erikson, Saab Military Aircraft
Robert Hillgren, Saab Military Aircraft
Lars Rundqwist, Saab Military Aircraft

The committee also benefited from a public lecture on March 4, 1996, by Professor A. V. Efremov, head of the pilot-vehicle laboratory at the Moscow Aviation Institute, during a visit to the United States. The lecture was attended by several committee members.

APPENDIX C

Details of Aircraft-Pilot Coupling Examples

This appendix provides quantitative details of the APC examples discussed in summary form in the body of the report.

ESSENTIALLY LINEAR OSCILLATORY AIRCRAFT-PILOT COUPLING EVENTS

The simplest oscillatory APC events occur when both the effective aircraft and the pilot dynamics act as quasi-linear and time-stationary system elements. In terms of the pilot behavioral modes described in Chapter 5, the pilot dynamic behavior associated with the instability is initially compensatory but may change to synchronous as the oscillation becomes fully developed.

Figures C-1a and C-1b show the pitch attitude characteristics of an illustrative set of effective aircraft dynamics tested in flight and extensively analyzed.[5,42] If it is assumed that the pilot operates in synchronous (pure gain) mode at the frequencies of interest, then data in Figures C-1a and C-1b correspond to the open-loop pilot-vehicle system (PVS) dynamics for pilot control using pitch attitude cues.

The key effective aircraft factors associated with susceptibility to an essentially linear PIO are properties that hinder the pilot's ability to close the PVS loop for various levels of pilot gain or to achieve adequate closed-loop performance. The first of these factors is illustrated by comparing Figures C-1a and C-1b. These are Bode plots and gain/phase (Nichols) diagrams of the open-loop dynamics of pilot-aircraft pitch attitude control systems.[43] Figure C-1a shows that a pure-gain pilot operating on attitude cues can create stable loop closures using gains from zero to a value somewhat less than the value

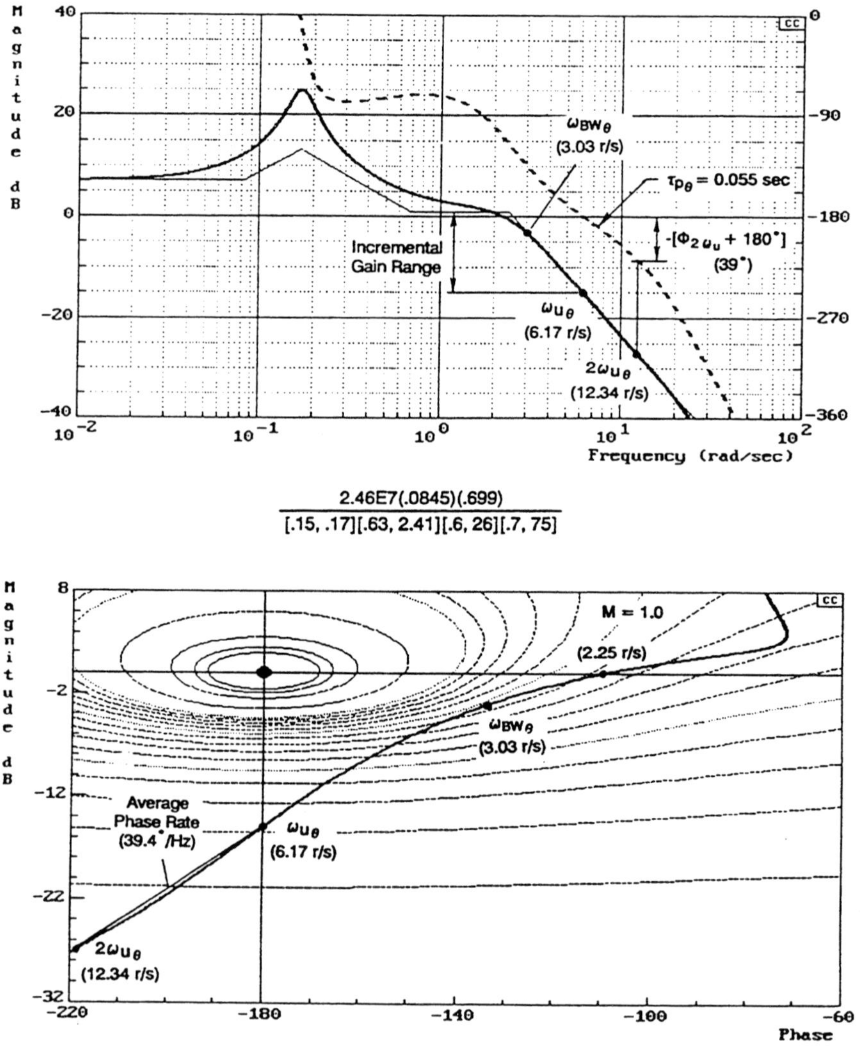

Baseline Configuration: 2-1 Pilot Ratings: 2/2/3 ; PIOR: 1/1/1 ; τ_p = 0.054 sec
Incremental Gain Range = 15.96 dB (6.28)

FIGURE C-1a Bode and Nichols diagrams for a synchronous PVS of an aircraft with low susceptibility to oscillatory APC events. Source: McRuer.[42]

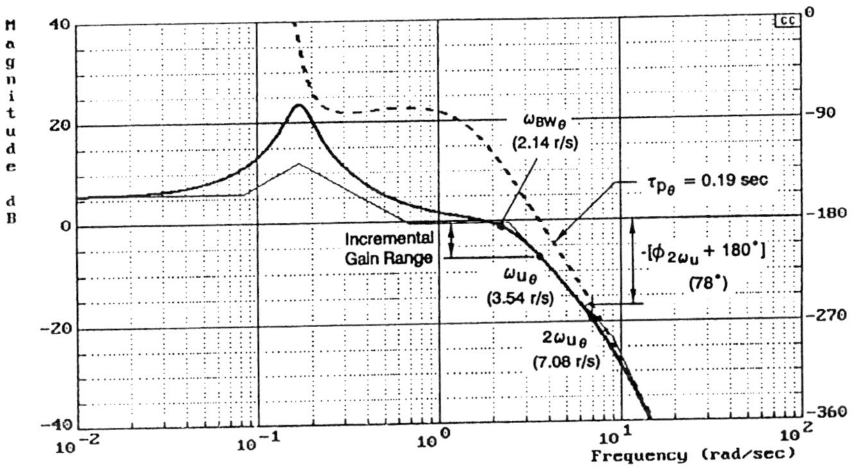

$$\frac{1.72E9(.0845)(.699)}{[.15,\ .17][.63,\ 2.41][.6,\ 26][.7,\ 75]} \quad \frac{1}{(.7,\ 9)}$$

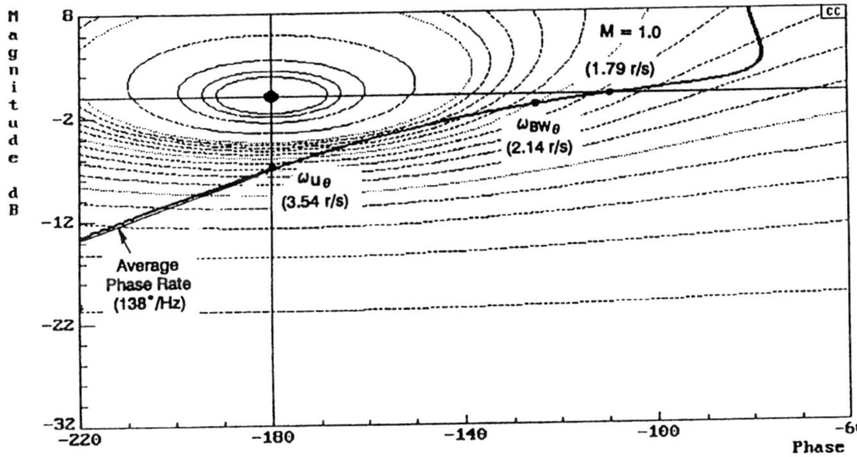

Configuration: 2-8 {2-1 ∗ 1/[.7,9]} Pilot Ratings: 8/10/8 ; PIOR: 4/4/4 ; τ_p = 0.19 sec
Incremental Gain Range = 6.60 dB (2.14)

FIGURE C-1b Bode and Nichols diagrams for a synchronous PVS of an aircraft with high susceptibility to oscillatory APC events. Source: McRuer.[42]

corresponding to the neutral stability frequency, ω_u (6.17 rad/sec), where the pilot-effective aircraft open-loop phase angle is −180 degrees. Within this entire range, the pilot can adjust gain as needed to achieve a desired level of closed-loop performance and control precision. Contrast this with the PVS attitude dynamics of Figure C-1b, where the maximum stable open-loop gain yields a neutral stability frequency of only 3.54 rad/sec. Because closed-loop system bandwidth and precision control (error performance) is proportional to the open-loop system gain, the attainable performance for the Figure C-1a system will be 1.75 times better than for the Figure C-1b system.

The analytically derived performance differences described above are reflected in the flight test experiments for these configurations.[5] The Cooper-Harper Pilot Rating (CH PR) differences (2/2/3 versus 8/10/8) from the flight tests show that the flying qualities of the Figure C-1a aircraft are excellent while those of the Figure C-1b configuration are terrible. The PIO rating differences (1/1/1 versus 4/4/4) further indicate the high susceptibility of the latter aircraft to PIO, which was aptly demonstrated when several PIOs were encountered.[5]

The extent to which the pilot can adjust gain in tight closed-loop control circumstances is measured by the "incremental gain adjustment range."[42] This feature can be quantified in various ways. For instance it could be expressed as a frequency range—for example, from 0 to 3.54 rad/sec and from 0 to 6.17 rad/sec for the characteristics compared above. Or, when a suitable reference level exists, it could be expressed in terms of an incremental pilot gain. For those effective aircraft dynamics where a short period "shelf" exists (the horizontal asymptote starts at $1/T_{\theta 2}$ = 0.7 rad/sec in Figures C-1a and C-1b and runs horizontally until it reaches the short-period, ω_{sp} = 2.41 rad/sec), the amplitude ratio of the shelf asymptote can serve as a convenient and relevant reference gain level, as noted in the figures (relevant because, for the pilot to exert significant control over the effective short period dynamics of the effective aircraft, the minimum open-loop system gain crossover has to be somewhat greater than this value). An analysis of the several severe aircraft pilot coupling oscillations (Figure C-1b, for example) indicates that an available gain range from this kind of reference should be greater than a factor of 3 (9.5 dB) or so to avoid a high degree of susceptibility to essentially linear severe APC oscillations.[5,42] In the example in Figure C-1b, it is only 6.6 dB. This same feature is implicitly reflected in indicators of K/s-like character, such as the Dropback criterion (see Chapter 6).

The inability to achieve adequate closed-loop system performance is also illustrated by Figures C-1a and C-1b when considered in the context of the associated pilot ratings. Achieving adequate performance with a linear system can be interpreted as attaining a specific open-loop system crossover frequency (ω_c). In terms of the aircraft dynamics, the attainable crossover frequency without extensive pilot compensation is conveniently measured by the so-called aircraft bandwidth (ω_{BW}). In this situation, the aircraft bandwidth is the frequency at which the phase is −135 degrees. The pilot ratings suggest that the ω_{BW} = 3.03 rad/sec for the Figure C-1a aircraft is excellent, while the Figure C-1b system ω_{BW} = 2.14 rad/sec is deficient.

The aircraft bandwidth can also be used as a basis for assessing the latitude available to the pilot in tightly closing the PVS loop. This basis contrasts the bandwidth frequency, as a nominal high-gain pilot-vehicle crossover frequency, with the maximum frequency available (ω_u). The incremental frequency ($\Delta\omega = \omega_u - \omega_{BW}$) indicates the maximum increase in crossover frequency from the aircraft bandwidth that is available from an increase in pilot gain. As a dimensionless scalar measure, $\Delta\omega / \omega_{BW}$ does much the same thing. For the contrasting "good" (Figure C-1a) and "bad" (Figure C-1b) aircraft, respectively, these parameters are $\Delta\omega$ = 3.14 rad/sec and 1.4 rad/sec and $\Delta\omega/\omega_{BW}$ = 1.04 and 0.65. Thus the pilot has much greater latitude to increase the open-loop system bandwidth, thereby improving both performance and accuracy, with the good aircraft of Figure C-1a.

The aircraft bandwidth is an excellent absolute indicator of the capability of a PVS for precision closed-loop control. The flexibility and ease of making precision adjustments, assessed via various available gain range measures, as above, often have arbitrary reference levels. They are, therefore, useful for comparing specific related configurations, such as the two aircraft in these examples, but cannot easily be used to generalize across unrelated configurations. A more general way to assess this feature is to examine the rapidity of change in the aircraft phase in the region of extremely tight control near the limiting maximum available frequency (ω_u). A convenient indicator for this purpose is available from many flying qualities studies. This is the "phase delay" (τ_{p9}) which measures the rate of change of phase lag based on the instability frequency (see Chapter 6). For the data in Figure C-1a and C-1b, these are 0.054 sec and 0.19 sec, respectively. In terms of all the criteria for flying qualities, the C-1a configuration is consistent with excellent Level 1, while the C-1b configuration is, at best, borderline PIO-prone.

All of the problems in the Figure C-1b system are direct consequences of the significantly greater high-frequency phase lag. Indeed, excessive lag is the most profoundly important single factor in essentially linear APC events because it limits both the attainable gain range and the attainable crossover frequency. The phase delay or some related quantity, such as average phase rate, and the aircraft bandwidth (ω_{BW}) are excellent summary indicators of the properties of the effective controlled element dynamics in closed-loop control.

SOME NONLINEAR CHARACTERISTICS THAT CAN LEAD TO FLYING QUALITIES CLIFFS

Common Cliff Producers

Conceptually, the cliff metaphor evokes a picture of sudden large changes in aircraft motions associated with relatively slight changes in pilot activity. When cliff-like changes are caused only by an increase in the pilot's output amplitude, the pilot-aircraft system is not behaving like a linear system. Instead, there are significant nonlinearities in the dynamics of either the effective aircraft or the pilot.

In conventional mechanical/hydraulic manual primary flight control systems (FCSs), the principal nonlinearities are rate and position limits intrinsic to surface actuators and various preloads, thresholds, and detents. These latter features are introduced to offset frictional and other unfavorable effects, thereby improving the threshold properties of the cockpit manipulators. In other words, they are intended to make the primary mechanical control system feel more "linear." Thus, in a well designed mechanical system, the significant nonlinearities involved in tightly controlled closed-loop control are the rate and position of the surface actuator.

By contrast, fly-by-wire (FBW) FCSs offer a more extensive variety of possibilities for deliberate nonlinearities. These opportunities are often fully exploited, although not always with a comprehensive understanding and appreciation of the accompanying side effects, not the least of which can be an enhanced susceptibility to APC events. Some simple examples are described below.

Perhaps the two most common significant nonlinear characteristics within the effective aircraft are present in the FCS. These are command-path gain-shaping and rate limiting. Figure 2-2 (see Chapter 2) shows a simplified view of these nonlinearities in a FCS/aircraft ("effective aircraft") combination. Note that rate limiters can be present in several different locations. However, just as with the primary manual control systems of the past, one source of rate limiting illustrated in Figures 2-2 and 2-3 is in the fully-powered surface actuating subsystem. This limiting rate is still around, although it is sometimes "protected" from becoming active by pre-actuator rate limiters. In this example, a pre-actuation-loop rate limiter or a rate limiter intrinsic to the actuation system will have the same effect. Command-path gain-shaping and rate limiting are used in the two elementary examples below to illustrate the cliff-like APC potential that can be introduced.

Command-Path Gain-Shaping

Most modern FCSs incorporate gain-shaping in the pilot's command path. The shaping is usually shallow around neutral, with the gain (control gradients) adjusted to provide optimum pilot-aircraft closed-loop precision control. In Figure 2-4, this is the region $|A| < a$. For larger pilot-input amplitudes, the gradient(s) are increased at points along the gain curve (e.g., at $A = a$) until maximum deflection of the control effector is achieved by maximum pilot input. (It should be noted in passing that the abrupt change in slope at $|A| = a$ is often made more smoothly and gradually.)

A typical PIO scenario involving this nonlinear feature might start with the PVS operating with high gain to achieve precision control around neutral. In terms of Figures 2-2 and 2-4 (see Chapter 2), the pilot's amplitude (A) for this condition does not exceed (a), although it can be arbitrarily close. To achieve a high degree of precision control, the pilot will be closing the loop with a relatively low gain margin. (Gain margin is the ratio of the open-loop system gain for instability to the operating point gain. In a typical PVS engaged in a high-gain tracking task, experimental data indicate that the gain margin will be nominally about 3/2 or 3.5 dB.[45] In this case, an increase in the open-loop system gain, from either the pilot or the effective aircraft, of 50 per cent would result in neutral stability.)

If a large input or disturbance, or even greater task demands, result in a pilot output amplitude of $|A| > a$, the effective open-loop gain of the PVS will increase. If the increase is sufficient to consume the gain margin, then a PIO can occur. Figure C-2 shows the stability limits for a gain margin of 3/2 as a function of the gain-shaping slope ratio. The robust stability limit for any K_2/K_1 is given by the initial abscissa (i.e., $\Delta G_M = 3/2$ for $a/A = 0$). For values of the slope ratio $K_2/K_1 > 1.5$ there will be an input amplitude (A) that gives rise to an oscillatory instability once it is exceeded.

A typical moderate value of K_2/K_1 is about 3, although higher values do exist. For the high-gain PVS closure assumed here, an oscillation will occur for any pilot input amplitude over (4/3)a, or only a 33 per cent increase in the input amplitude beyond the slope break-upward point. Gains that are similarly sensitive to the pilot input have been indicted as a source of PIOs in the past, including the YF-22 case described in Chapter 2 and by James et al.[36] Input-sensitive gains can act independently or in concert with various rate limiting features to cause an APC event.

Rate Limiting

Extensive control-surface rate limiting has been observed in almost all recorded severe oscillatory APC events. Detailed analyses of rate limiting support the view that rate limiting exacerbates time lag effects.[3,14,15,28,31,39] But how and when the additional time lags enter the closed-loop system have not been well documented in detailed experiments.

Although there is a consensus that rate limiting phenomena are important factors in fully developed, severe APC events encountered in operational situations, the transitional system behavior on the way to rate limiting and severe PVS oscillations has not been recorded in enough detail for a complete understanding. The possibility that rate limiting phenomena may be central initiating factors (triggers) in the development of some severe APC events has also not received enough attention. Yet it is easy to show that rate limiting features in FCSs can lead to unusual, potentially cliff-like situations.

Some general aspects of rate limiting in actuation systems are described in the discussion of Figure 2-3 (see Chapter 2). When the input frequencies (PIO frequencies) are much smaller than the bandwidth of the actuation system, these rate limiting features can be generalized as properties of a "rate-limiting element." Actuator rate limiting characteristics that do not rely on this simplifying assumption have been developed.[39] Both the time-domain and frequency-domain properties of a rate-limiting element are shown in Figure C-3.

Figure C-3a shows the output of the rate limiting element to a sinusoidal input as a triangular wave. This will occur when the system input amplitude (A) and input frequency (ω) create a maximum input-velocity command (ωA)

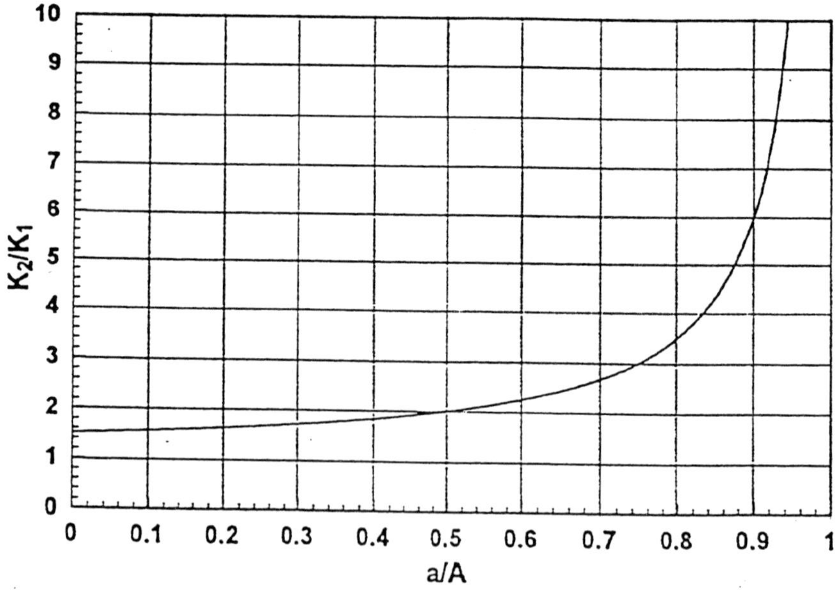

FIGURE C-2 Input amplitude-dependent stability boundaries as a function of command-path gain shaping ratio for a linear system gain margin $\Delta G_M = 1.5$.

large enough to keep the system essentially always on the rate limit. Figure C-3b gives a describing function for the amplitude ratio and phase angle as functions of a frequency ratio in which the normalizing frequency is the "onset frequency" (ω_{ON}). At the onset frequency, the input rate equals the rate limit (i.e., $\omega_{ON} A = V_L$, where A is the amplitude of the input position command and V_L is the rate limit).

At normalized frequencies (ω/ω_{ON}) less than one, the amplitude ratio of the rate-limiting element is 1.0 and the phase lag is zero. Thus rate limiting, as expected, has no effect whatsoever in this range. At and slightly above the onset frequency, the amplitude ratio decreases somewhat, and a phase lag begins. This is the "transition" or "near saturation" zone (see Figure C-3b). Finally, when input amplitudes are large enough (or rate limits small enough) to pass the fully-developed onset frequency ($\omega_{ON-FD} = 1.862\ \omega_{ON}$), the rate limiting becomes fully developed, introducing a significant phase lag into the PVS loop.[14] This condition can lead to a cliff-like situation because the insertion of the phase lag occurs simultaneously with the increase in the magnitude of the pilot's command. At its most insidious, the phenomenon causes the sudden and dramatic onset of a substantial shift in the phase lag. This shift is equivalent to the sudden insertion of a significant added time delay into the loop.

A typical scenario might begin with a pilot who is well-adapted to an essentially linear closed-loop PVS that is operating at high gain to satisfy precision control purposes. The system is then confronted with task demands that call for just a bit more pilot control amplitude or gain. When the system is near the conditions for the onset of rate limiting, slight increases in either amplitude or gain (or both) are sufficient to enter the non-linear rate-limiting regions, with the concomitant introduction of a sudden substantial phase lag into the closed-loop system. (Recall the F-14 example described in Chapter 2.) In terms of the underlying physics of closed-loop systems, this is a classic example of jump resonance.[28]

To illustrate the general points about jump resonance and flying qualities cliffs caused by rate limiting in more quantitative detail, consider a closed-loop control task with effective aircraft dynamics that possesses nominally excellent flying qualities and to which the pilot is well-adapted. The PVS dynamics in the linear regime will be approximated by the crossover model of manual control theory. Assume that the effective vehicle dynamics include a rate-limited actuator operating in series with the pilot and that the effective aircraft in the linear regime possesses excellent flying qualities. When task demands require tight closed-loop performance, the pilot's gain and maximum amplitude are adjusted to satisfy the precision control requirements. Assume that these levels remain consistent with linear system operations, but with rate limit/pilot-input-amplitude values near the onset (or saturation) frequency. With an active,

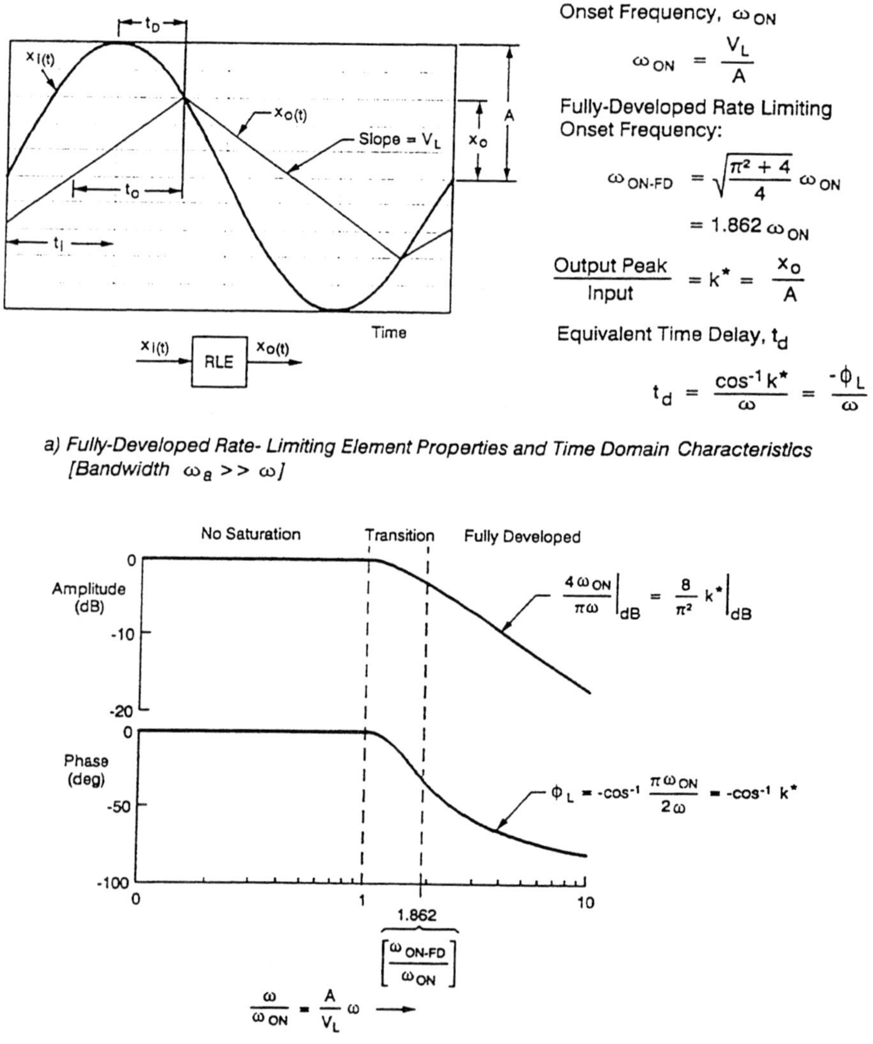

FIGURE C-3 Time domain and transfer characteristics for fully developed rate limiting.

attentive pilot, this baseline condition would exhibit a gain margin of about 3/2 and a phase margin of perhaps 25 degrees. In this essentially linear regime, the closed-loop system will perform well. It would be given Level 1 flying qualities assessments with good CH PRs and low PIO ratings and would exhibit no significant periodic oscillations.

Now increase the task demands so that the pilot's input amplitude is increased by 10 to 20 percent. This can be enough to push the system well past the onset frequency to a point where the phase margin is reduced from about 25 degrees to zero, resulting in a potentially severe PIO. With just a bit more input amplitude, the rate limiting can become fully active, introducing a much greater phase lag and a diverging closed-loop system oscillation.

To make this example even more specific, assume that the effective aircraft dynamics are consistent with excellent pilot ratings—say a CH PR of 2 or 3. For this to be so, the effective time delay (τ_e in the crossover model—which accounts for both the pilot's lags and the higher-frequency dynamics of the effective aircraft) will be about 0.3 sec. In this crossover model case, the neutral stability frequency ($\omega_u = \pi/2\ \tau_e$) will be about 5 rad/sec, which is representative of the linear system.[39,42] Taking the 25 degrees phase lag caused by rate limiting into account, the PIO frequency becomes about 3.5 rad/sec. This PIO frequency is 30 percent less than the neutral stability frequency of 5 rad/sec for the linear system. The sudden phase lag introduced by the phase deficit of 25 degrees can then, with the known PIO frequency, be equated to an equivalent incremental time lag of 0.12 sec. Thus, the frequency of the PIO is the same as would occur if an incremental delay of t_d = 0.12 sec was suddenly inserted into the system.

For the effective aircraft to have excellent flying qualities initially, the effective time delay of the aircraft alone would be about 0.1 sec or so, which would be more than doubled by virtue of the rate limiting effect. The total effective delay of 0.22 sec for the nonlinear system is also well above the value of about 0.19 sec associated with a high degree of PIO susceptibility for a linear system.

McRuer et al[46] have provided a more detailed and precise analysis of these rate-limiting and gain-shaping effects. The examples above illustrate the importance of nonlinear concepts for identifying rate limiting and kindred features as potential sources of nonlinear, oscillatory, jump-resonance phenomena. The jump-resonance phenomenon is useful because it exhibits nonlinear features that correspond well with test pilot descriptions of nonlinear, cliff-like behavior when severe APC events occur (see Chapter 2).

APPENDIX D

Research

ONGOING AIRCRAFT-PILOT COUPLING SIMULATION TECHNIQUE RESEARCH

A critical technical tool in the design and development of new or modified aircraft is the piloted simulator. These include in-flight simulators and ground-based simulators with varying degrees of sophistication, from simple piloted combat stations ("work stations") to high fidelity, wide field-of-view facilities with large-amplitude motion base capability. (For a discussion of the necessary considerations for using these facilities, see Chapter 5.) In general, the current simulation techniques have been inadequate for exposing APC characteristics prior to flight tests. The purpose of this appendix is to describe current research to improve piloted simulator capabilities in APC evaluations.

T-33 Have PIO Simulation Technique

One current research project is an evaluation of the relative effectiveness of ground-based piloted simulator equipment with varying degrees of sophistication. Using "best engineering practices" to model the T-33 APC flight test experiment (called "Have PIO"), the research project focuses on variations of parameters in the longitudinal aircraft axis that influence PIO events. Piloted evaluations are then conducted on each type of facility: the Large Amplitude Multimode Aerospace Research Simulator (LAMARS) with and without motion; the MS-1 (40-foot visual dome); and the Piloted Combat Station. Pilot ratings, both Cooper-Harper Pilot Ratings and PIO ratings, are recorded for each configuration and compared with flight tests. Subsequent changes can be made to the simulation model, facility, task, or pilot stress level to try to improve upon comparisons to flight tests. These experiments will identify the most reliable adjusted simulation techniques for exposing linear APC tendencies during landing for fighter applications. This project is scheduled to be completed in the second quarter of fiscal year 1997.

C-17 Comparison between In-Flight and Ground-Based Simulation and Flight Test

Another more sophisticated research study on the development of simulation techniques has just been initiated to evaluate and compare piloted simulation capabilities for exposing APC tendencies on transport aircraft. First, the C-17 high fidelity, motion-based simulator will be used to evaluate APC tendencies with degraded flight control changes. The specific flying tasks, emergency procedures, and APC events will be systematically defined and recorded. Then, the C-17 development test aircraft, T1, with its Change-A-Gain system, will be used to force APC events to occur in a safe manner during the APC flight test tasks identified on the simulator. The results will be compared and changes made to the simulation process, as required, to maximize agreement between flight tests and the ground-based simulations. Finally, the simulation experiment will be repeated using the Total In-Fight Simulator (TIFS) aircraft to evaluate the effectiveness of in-flight simulation in exposing APC characteristics. This project will require a minimum of 20 months to complete; T1 flight testing is planned for the first quarter of fiscal year 1997, and TIFS flight testing is planned for the second quarter of fiscal year 1997.

Development of APC Simulation Techniques for Fighter Aircraft Using the Variable Stability In-Flight Simulator Test Aircraft

A research experiment similar to the C-17 project is planned for fighter-type aircraft in fiscal year 1998. A similar approach to the one outlined above is planned using the F-16 Variable Stability In-Flight Simulator Test Aircraft (VISTA). Unique APC simulation techniques for maximizing simulator effectiveness will be developed.

APC COMPENSATION AND DETECTION RESEARCH

Compensation System Research

In the past, several attempts aimed solely at APC attenuation have been tried, with varying degrees of success. The general application of the proposed approaches has not been thoroughly investigated, and the inherent limitations resulting from limiting phase lag and frequency bandwidth parameters to keep APC events from occurring must still be studied. Rather than attempting to detect APC tendencies, these studies focus on preventing the buildup of phase lag or filtering high frequency control inputs. The filter approach is currently used on the space shuttle.[58] Phase lag compensation has shown some promise in preventing rate-limit-induced APC events.[1,10,41] The extent to which this approach may limit desired maneuverability for otherwise APC-free maneuvers has not been adequately investigated. An approach like this has been incorporated into the Swedish Gripen (JAS 39) control system.[60] Parameter compensation techniques coupled with a highly reliable detection system may provide a good integrated approach that would not limit maneuverability until an APC event is detected or extreme values of key APC-related parameters have been exceeded without APC detection.

Development of Theory-Based Detection Algorithm

As part of an integrated research effort to develop APC-resistant design criteria and development processes, a set of theory-based engineering algorithms is being developed that will provide on-board early detection of incipient APC events. Subsequent efforts will result in a complete system design that defines the detailed components, from sensor signal to warning device or compensation. A complete system will be developed and validated on current aircraft. Emphasis will be placed on minimizing unnecessary warnings and compensation while minimizing the occurrence of APC events.

Neural Network Empirically-Based Detection System

A completely different approach to on-board detection and compensation is being investigated using data from current APC events to train a neural network. The resulting algorithms will not require that the theory be developed in advance of an effective solution. The trained neural network will recognize and distinguish APC events before they become unmanageable. Initial trials of a relatively crude, single-axis neural network were very promising on the limited number of APC events tested. It should be noted that these early test cases included neural network identification of a nonlinear APC event on an F-18 aircraft even though the network was trained on F-16 linear APC events. Much work still needs to be done to train the network on a sufficient number of APC events to make this approach effective for all types of aircraft and APC events. After detection algorithms have been developed, substantial efforts will be required to verify and validate that the network is effective and safe. The precise compensation required once an incipient APC event is identified will also need to be evaluated.

Acronyms

APC	aircraft-pilot coupling
CH PR	Cooper-Harper Pilot Rating
FAA	Federal Aviation Administration
FBW	fly-by-wire
FCS	flight control system
FDR	flight data recorder
FMS	flight management system
FOQA	Flight Operational Quality Assurance
HQDT	handling qualities during tracking
NASA	National Aeronautics and Space Administration
NRC	National Research Council
NTSB	National Transportation Safety Board
OCM	optimal control model
PIO	pilot-involved (or pilot-induced) oscillation
PVS	pilot-vehicle system
QAR	quick access recorder
SAS	stability augmentation system

Glossary

The following technical terms are not defined in the report and may be unfamiliar to some readers.

Aircraft bandwidth (ω_{bw}). A measure of the range of frequencies over which a pilot can exert good closed-loop control without excessive compensation (e.g., excessive pilot lead or anticipation). At the nominal aircraft attitude to controller input (θ/δ_p) bandwidth frequency, ω_{bw_θ}, the θ/δ_p phase angle is -135° (see Figure 6-1).

Amplitude ratio. The ratio of the amplitudes of the steady-state output and input when the input is a sine wave. This ratio is often expressed in decibels (dB) where $[\text{amplitude ratio}]_{dB} = 20 \log_{10} x$ [amplitude ratio].

Bandwidth. A measure of the highest frequency sinusoidal input that a linear system can track with reasonable fidelity. Often defined as the frequency where the amplitude ratio of the system is 3 dB below the zero frequency value.

Bobweight effect. The overall effect of unbalanced masses (bobweights) intrinsic to or deliberately introduced into various locations throughout a mechanical control system. Bobweight effect can serve the positive purpose of providing cues to the pilot regarding accelerations of the aircraft.

Bode diagram. A Bode diagram presents system transfer function or frequency response data plotted in rectangular coordinate form. The amplitude ratio (output-to-input) expressed in dB and phase angle are plotted against frequency on a log scale.

Buffet. Buffet refers to the unsteady aircraft motion caused by flow conditions over parts of the aircraft, typically during transonic flight or low-speed conditions preceding a stall.

C*U integrator. "C*U" is the popular name for a particular pitch axis control law that Boeing uses in the flight control system of the 777. As seen in Figure 2-10, the C*U integrator provides a feedback signal that incorporates pitch rate, normal acceleration, speed error, and column position. Thus, in steady state, column commands result in an incremental speed change. The other terms in the C*U signal are combined with the column feed forward and pitch rate signals to provide the desired effective aircraft dynamics.

Carefree flight. A type of flying in which the pilot is free to maneuver the aircraft in a "carefree" manner with little or no concern for particular task constraints. Carefree flying can be an exploratory experiment to discover latent, unanticipated APC susceptibilities.

Cliff. The "cliff" metaphor is used to convey a sense of unexpected, dramatic, and excessively large changes in aircraft motion associated with relatively slight changes in pilot activity. When cliff-like changes result from an incremental increase in the amplitude of the pilot's output, the pilot-vehicle system is not behaving like a linear system. Instead, this indicates the presence of significant nonlinearities either in the dynamics of the effective aircraft or in the pilot's behavior. Many, if not all, Category II and III PIOs exhibit cliff-like behavior.

Closed-loop feedback system. A combination of control system elements in which command variables are compared with desired output variables. If the outputs differ from the desired values, corrective signals are sent to control actuating elements to bring the controlled variables to their proper values.

Cooper-Harper Pilot Rating (CH PR). A numerical flying (or handling) qualities rating (1–10) a pilot assigns to an aircraft and piloting task that indicates the workload the task required and the performance that could be obtained. A rating of 1 indicates optimum handling qualities.

Divergence. An unstable system response characterized by an output of increasing amplitude when the input, itself, is bounded. Divergences are associated with aperiodic (non-oscillatory) APC events.

Flight envelope. The bounds within which a certain flight system can operate, especially a graphic representation of these bounds showing the interrelationships of operational parameters.

Flight management computer. A computerized system found in the cockpits of modern commercial aircraft that can automate many of the tasks normally performed by the pilot. These tasks include route planning, navigation, fuel management, and aircraft control.

Fly-by-light. A control system that uses optoelectronic systems to transmit control information by light through fiber-optic cables.
Fly-by-wire. A control system that uses conventional electronic systems to transmit control information via electrical cables.
Flying qualities. Aircraft characteristics that govern the ease or precision with which the pilot can accomplish specific tasks.
Frequency response. The response of a component, instrument, or control system to input signals at varying frequencies. For example, the frequency response characteristics of a servoactuator are defined as the steady-state relationship of the output amplitude to the input amplitude and the output-to-input phase difference when the input is subjected to constant amplitude sinusoidal signals of various frequencies.

Gain. In general, the ratio of output to input of a control system element. For elements with low-pass filter-like characteristics, gain is the amplitude ratio at zero frequency. **Pilot gain** is the sensitivity with which the pilot reacts to a given percept. If the situation is urgent, the pilot is likely to react with large corrective inputs even for small system errors. When this happens, the pilot is said to be exhibiting high gain. More relaxed responses imply a lower pilot gain.

Handling qualities. See flying qualities.

Limit. See "rate limit" and "position limit."
Limit cycle. The name given to a system oscillation in which the frequency and amplitude are determined by the nonlinear properties of the system.

Neuromuscular system. The system that governs human movement, generally consisting of nerves (neuro-), which provide commands and feedback from and to the central nervous system, and muscles (-muscular), which generate the forces necessary for movement.

Peak magnification ratio. The maximum amplitude ratio for a system determined across all input frequencies.
Phase lag. The phase difference between the input and output of a system in which the input is a sine wave. The "lag" applies when the output, or response, lags in time behind the input or command.
Phase margin. A measure of system stability defined as the phase lag to be added to achieve 180° of phase lag at the open-loop frequency response corresponding to the 0 dB amplitude ratio.
Pipper. A small symbol, typically a circle or square, that appears in the gun sight (head-up display) of a fighter aircraft indicating pointing errors between

the target and the chase aircraft. Pipper errors are typically described in terms of angular displacement such as "mils" (milliradians).
Position limit. The maximum allowable deflection for an aircraft control surface or other effector, based on either mechanical limits associated with the actuation system or on lower limits imposed by the flight control system.
Proprioceptive. Perceptions of forces and movements of the pilot's body (including limb).

Rate limit. The maximum allowable rate of deflection for an aircraft control surface or other effector, based on either the maximum rate at which the actuation system can reposition the control surface or on lower limits imposed by the flight control system.

Stability augmentation system (SAS). A subsystem of the flight control system that uses sensors, actuators, etc., to augment the basic dynamic properties of the aircraft. When considered as an entity, the SAS is essentially a closed-loop regulator control system. SAS signals are introduced in series with pilot inputs so the SAS signals do not cause stick motion or forces, but still serve to modify the effective aircraft dynamics. On older aircraft, the SAS generally has limited authority.

Upset. An upset refers to a sudden, large change in aircraft attitude that was not deliberately commanded by the pilot. Upsets are frequently caused by atmospheric turbulence.

Washout filters. Washout filters remove the low frequency components of commanded cab motion in moving-base simulators.
Workload. The total of the combined physical and mental demands upon a person.

References

[1]A'Harrah, R. 1994. An alternate control scheme for alleviating aircraft-pilot coupling. AIAA Paper No. 94-3673. Pp. 1194–1201 in Proceedings of the American Institute of Aeronautics and Astronautics (AIAA) Guidance, Navigation and Control Conference, Scottsdale, Arizona, August 1–3, 1994. Reston, Virginia: American Institute of Aeronautics and Astronautics (AIAA).

[2]Ad Hoc Advisory Subcommittee on Avionics, Controls, and Human Factors. 1979. Proposed Study of Simulation Validation/Fidelity for NASA Simulators. November 1979. Washington, D.C.: National Aeronautics and Space Administration.

[3]Ashkenas, I., H. Jex, and D. McRuer. 1964. Pilot Induced Oscillations: Their Causes and Analysis. Northrop-Norair Report NOR 64-143. Prepared by Systems Technology, Inc. Report STI TR-239-2. June 20, 1964.

[4]Bailey, R., and T. Bidlack. 1995. Unified Pilot-Induced Oscillation Theory. Vol. 4: Time-Domain Neal-Smith Criterion. Report No. WL-TR-96-3031. Wright-Patterson Air Force Base, Ohio: Wright Laboratory.

[5]Bjorkman, E. 1986. Flight Test Evaluation of Techniques to Predict Longitudinal Pilot Induced Oscillations. Thesis AFIT/GAE/AA/86J-1. Wright-Patterson Air Force Base, Ohio: Air Force Institute of Technology.

[6]Bode, W.H. 1945. Network Analysis and Feedback Amplifier Design. Princeton, New Jersey: Van Nostrand.

[7]Bouwer, G., A. Taghizad, and H. Moedden. 1996. Smart Helicopter Concept—Handling Qualities Data Base for Hover and Low Speed Flight. Paper presented at Advisory Group for Aerospace Research and Development (AGARD) Flight Vehicle Integration Panel Symposium on Advances in Rotorcraft Technology. Ottawa, Canada, May 1996. (Available from NASA Center for AeroSpace Information [CASI], 800 Elkridge Landing Road, Linthicum Heights, Maryland.)

[8]Buchacker, E., H. Galleithner, R. Koehler, and M. Marchand. 1990. Development of MIL-8785C into a Handling Qualities Specification for a New European Fighter Aircraft. Pp. 10–16 in Flying Qualities. Report No. AGARD-CP-508. Proceedings of Flight Mechanics Panel Symposium, Quebec City, Canada, October 15–18, 1990. (Available from NASA Center for AeroSpace Information [CASI], 800 Elkridge Landing Road, Linthicum Heights, Maryland.)

[9]Chalk, C. 1995. Calspan Experience of PIO and the Effects of Rate Limiting. Pp. 12-1–12-12 in Flight Vehicle Integration Panel Workshop on Pilot Induced Oscillations. Report No. AGARD-AR-335. (Available from NASA Center for AeroSpace Information [CASI], 800 Elkridge Landing Road, Linthicum Heights, Maryland.)

[10]Deppe, P.R. 1993. Flight Evaluation of a Software Rate Limiter Concept. Calspan Final Report No. 8091-1. Buffalo, New York: Calspan Advanced Technology Center.

[11]Dornheim, M. 1992. Report pinpoints factors leading to YF-22 crash. Aviation Week and Space Technology 137(19):53–54.

[12]Dornheim, M. 1995. Boeing corrects several 777 PIOs. Aviation Week and Space Technology 142(19):32–33.

[13]Dornheim, M. 1995. Dramatic incidents highlight mode problems in cockpits. Aviation Week and Space Technology 142(5):57–59.

[14]Duda, H. 1994. Berücksichtigung von Stellratenbegrenzern in Flugregelsystemen bei der Systembewertung im Frequenzbereich (Frequency Domain Analysis of Rate Limiting Elements in Flight Control Systems). Report No. DLR-FB 94-16. Braunschweig, Germany: Deutsche Forschungsanstalt für Luft- und Raumfahrt (DLR) Institut für Flugmechanik.

[15]Duda, H. 1995. Effects of Rate Limiting Elements in Flight Control Systems—A New PIO Criterion. AIAA Paper No. 95-3204. Pp. 288–298 in Proceedings of the AIAA Guidance, Navigation and Control Conference, Baltimore, Maryland, August 7–10, 1995. Reston, Virginia: AIAA.

[16]Duda, H. 1996. Open Loop Onset Point: A New Flying Qualities Parameter to Predict A-PC Problems due to Rate Saturation in FCS. Report No. DLR IB 111-96/1. Braunschweig, Germany: DLR Institut für Flugmechanik.

[17]Duda, H. 1996. Prediction of Adverse Aircraft-Pilot Coupling in the Roll Axis due to Rate Limiting in Flight Control Systems. Report No. DLR IB 111-96/13. Braunschweig, Germany: DLR Institut für Flugmechanik.

[18]Efremov, A. 1995. Analysis of Reasons for Pilot Induced Oscillation Tendency and Development of Criteria for Its Prediction. Contract SPC-94-4028. Moscow, Russia: Pilot-Vehicle Laboratory, Moscow Aviation Institute.

[19]Enhagen, J. 1996. The Klonk Method. Presentation to a delegation of the Committee on the Effects of Aircraft-Pilot Coupling on Flight Safety, at Linköping, Sweden, May 6, 1996.

[20]Fink, D. 1977. Orbiter experiences control problems. Aviation Week and Space Technology 107(2):16.

[21]Gibson, J. 1982. Piloted Handling Qualities Design Criteria for High Order Flight Control Systems in Criteria for Handling Qualities of Military Aircraft. Report No. AGARD-CP-333. (Available from NASA Center for AeroSpace Information [CASI], 800 Elkridge Landing Road, Linthicum Heights, Maryland.)

[22]Gibson, J. 1995. Definition, Understanding, and Design of Aircraft Handling Qualities. Report No. LR-756. Delft, Netherlands: Delft University of Technology.

[23]Gibson, J. 1995. Looking for the Simple PIO Model. Pp. 5-1–5-11 in Flight Vehicle Integration Panel Workshop on Pilot Induced Oscillations. Report No. AGARD-AR-335. (Available from NASA Center for AeroSpace Information [CASI], 800 Elkridge Landing Road, Linthicum Heights, Maryland.)

[24]Gibson, J. 1995. Prevention of PIO by Design. Pp. 2-1–2-12 in Active Control Technology: Applications and Lessons Learned. Report No. AGARD-CP-560. Proceedings of Flight Mechanics Panel Symposium, Turin, Italy, May 9–13, 1994. (Available from NASA Center for AeroSpace Information [CASI], 800 Elkridge Landing Road, Linthicum Heights, Maryland.)

[25]Gibson, J. 1996. Personal communication to Duane McRuer, Committee on the Effects of Aircraft-Pilot Coupling on Flight Safety.

[26]Givens, M. 1994. Evaluation of B-2 Susceptibility to Pilot-Induced Oscillations. White Paper 120-4. Pico Rivera, California: Northrop Grumman, B-2 Division.

[27]Graham, D. 1967. Research on the Effect of Nonlinearities on Tracking Performance. Report No. AMRL-TR-67-9. Wright-Patterson Air Force Base, Ohio: Aerospace Medical Research Laboratories

[28]Graham, D., and D. McRuer. 1961. Analysis of Nonlinear Control Systems. New York: Reprinted by Dover, 1971.

[29]Hamel, P. 1996. Recent and Future Aircraft-Pilot Coupling Research at DLR. Report No. IB 111-96/15. Braunschweig, Germany: DLR Institut für Flugmechanik.

[30]Hamel, P. 1996. Rotorcraft-Pilot Coupling: A Critical Issue for Highly Augmented Helicopters? AGARD-CP-592. AGARD Symposium on Advances in Rotorcraft Technology, Ottawa, Canada, May 1996. (Available from NASA Center for AeroSpace Information [CASI], 800 Elkridge Landing Road, Linthicum Heights, Maryland.)

[31]Hanke, D. 1995. Handling qualities analysis on rate limiting elements in flight control systems. Pp. 11-1–11-18 in Flight Vehicle Integration Panel Workshop on Pilot Induced Oscillations. Report No. AGARD-AR-335. (Available from NASA Center for AeroSpace Information [CASI], 800 Elkridge Landing Road, Linthicum Heights, Maryland.)

[32]Harris, J. 1996. Personal communication from J. Harris, Lockheed Martin, to C. Droste, Committee on the Effects of Aircraft-Pilot Coupling on Flight Safety.

[33]Hess, R. 1983. A model-based investigation of manipulator characteristics and pilot/vehicle performance. Journal of Guidance, Control, and Dynamics 6(5): 348–354.

[34]Hess, R. 1996. Feedback control models—manual control and tracking. Chapter 38 in Handbook of Human Factors and Ergonomics. G. Salvendy (ed). New York: John Wiley and Sons.

[35]Hirsch, D., and R. McCormick. 1966. Experimental investigation of pilot dynamics in a pilot-induced oscillation situation. Journal of Aircraft 3(Nov–Dec):567–573.

[36]James, H., N. Nichols, and R. Phillips. 1947. Theory of Servomechanisms. New York: McGraw-Hill.

[37]Johnston, D., and D. McRuer. 1986. Investigation of Interactions Between Limb-Manipulator Dynamics and Effective Vehicle Roll Control Characteristics. Report

No. NASA CR-3983. Washington, D.C.: National Aeronautics and Space Administration.

[38]Kendall, E. 1995. C-17 Flying Qualities and Aircraft-Pilot Coupling (APC) Experience During the Development Process. Report No. MDC 96K7012. Long Beach, California: McDonnell Douglas.

[39]Klyde, D., D. McRuer, and T. Myers. 1995. Unified Pilot-Induced Oscillation Theory. Vol. I: PIO Analysis with Linear and Nonlinear Effective Vehicle Characteristics, Including Rate Limiting. Report No. WL-TR 96-3028. Wright-Patterson Air Force Base, Ohio: Wright Laboratory.

[40]Kullberg, E., and P. Elgcrona. 1995. Saab experience with PIO. Pp. 9-1–9-9 in Flight Vehicle Integration Panel Workshop on Pilot Induced Oscillations. Report No. AGARD-AR-335. (Available from NASA Center for AeroSpace Information [CASI], 800 Elkridge Landing Road, Linthicum Heights, Maryland.)

[41]Martin, J., and J. Buchholz. 1995. SCARLET: DLR rate saturation flight experiment. Pp. 8-1–8-6 in Flight Vehicle Integration Panel Workshop on Pilot Induced Oscillations. Report No. AGARD-AR-335. (Available from NASA Center for AeroSpace Information [CASI], 800 Elkridge Landing Road, Linthicum Heights, Maryland.)

[42]McRuer, D. 1995. Pilot-Induced Oscillations and Human Dynamic Behavior. NASA Contractor Report 4683. Washington, D.C.: National Aeronautics and Space Administration.

[43]McRuer, D., I. Ashkenas, and D. Graham. 1973. Aircraft Dynamics and Automatic Control. Princeton, New Jersey: Princeton University Press.

[44]McRuer, D., and E. Krendel. 1974. Mathematical Models of Human Pilot Behavior. Report No. AGARDograph 188. (Available from NASA Center for AeroSpace Information [CASI], 800 Elkridge Landing Road, Linthicum Heights, Maryland.)

[45]McRuer, D., W. Clement, P. Thompson, and R. Magdaleno. 1990. Pilot Modeling for Flying Qualities Applications. Vol. 2 of Minimum Flying Qualities. Report No. WRDC-TR-89-3125. Wright-Patterson Air Force Base, Ohio: Air Force Flight Dynamics Laboratory.

[46]McRuer, D., D. Klyde, and T. Myers. 1996. Development of a comprehensive PIO theory. AIAA Paper No. 96-3433. Pp. 581–597 in Proceedings of the AIAA Atmospheric Flight Mechanics Conference, San Diego, California, July 29–31, 1996. Reston, Virginia: AIAA.

[47]McWha, J. 1996. Personal communication from James McWha (Boeing) to the Committee on the Effects of Aircraft-Pilot Coupling on Flight Safety.

[48]Mitchell, D., and R. Hoh. 1995. Development of a Unified Method to Predict Tendencies for Pilot-Induced Oscillations. Report No. WL-TR-95-3049. Wright-Patterson Air Force Base, Ohio: Wright Laboratory.

[49]Mitchell, D., R. Hoh, B. Aponso, and D. Klyde. 1994. Proposed Incorporation of Mission-Oriented Flying Qualities into MIL STD-1797A. Report No. WL-TR-94-3162. Wright-Patterson Air Force Base, Ohio: Wright Laboratory.

[50]Moorehouse, D. 1995. YF-22 mishap and discussion of other PIOs. Presentation at the Workshop on Aircraft-Pilot Coupling, National Research Council, Irvine, California, November 27–29, 1995.

[51]National Transportation Safety Board (NTSB). 1995. Flight Data Recorder Factual Report of Investigation. Report No. CHI-95IA-138. Washington, D.C.: National Transportation Safety Board.

[52]NTSB. 1995. Safety Recommendation A-95-107 through -109. Washington, D.C.: National Transportation Safety Board.

[53]Neal, P., and R. Smith. 1970. An In-Flight Investigation to Develop Control System Design Criteria for Fighter Aircraft. Report No. AFFDL-TR-70-74, Vol. 1. Wright-Patterson Air Force Base, Ohio: Air Force Flight Dynamics Laboratory.

[54]Nelson, T., and R. Landes. 1996. Boeing 777 development and APC assessment. Presented at Society of Automotive Engineers (SAE) Control and Guidance Systems Conference, Salt Lake City, Utah, March 6–8, 1996. In press.

[55]Niewoehner, R. 1995. Probing APC Susceptibility through HQDT. Paper provided to the Committee on the Effects of Aircraft-Pilot Coupling on Flight Safety on December 22, 1995.

[56]Ockier, C. 1996. Pilot-Induced Oscillations in Helicopters—Three Case Studies. Report No. IB 111-96/12. Braunschweig, Germany: DLR Institut für Flugmechanik.

[57]Pitz, D. 1984. Report on the Heavy PIO Experienced with P13 during Terrain Following Investigations at E-61 Manching, Bundesamt für Wehrtechnik und Beschaffung (BWB), Ausgelagerter Fachbereich (AFB) bei der Erprobungsstelle 61 (E-61), Manching, AZ 11/84, 15 February 1984. Available from German Air Force Flight Test Center, Wehrtechnische Dienststelle für Luftfahrzeuge (WTD 61), Flugplatz, D-85077 Manching, Germany.

[58]Powers, B. 1982. An adaptive stick-gain to reduce pilot-induced oscillation tendencies. Journal of Guidance, Control, and Dynamics, 5 (March–April):138–142.

[59]Powers, B. 1984. Space Shuttle Pilot-Induced-Oscillation Research Testing. Report No. AGARDograph No. 262. In AGARD Ground and Flight Testing for Aircraft Guidance and Control (N85-22350 13-01). (Available from NASA Center for AeroSpace Information [CASI], 800 Elkridge Landing Road, Linthicum Heights, Maryland.)

[60]Rundqwist, L., and R. Hillgren. 1996. Phase compensation of rate limiters in JAS 39 Grippen. AIAA Paper No. 96-3368. Pp. 69–77 in Proceedings of the AIAA Atmospheric Flight Mechanics Conference, San Diego, California, July 29–31, 1996. Reston, Virginia: AIAA.

[61]Sekigawa, E., and M. Mecham, 1996. Pilots, A 300 systems cited in Nagoya crash. Aviation Week and Space Technology 145(5):36–37.

[62]Smith, J., and D. Berry. 1975. Analysis of Longitudinal Pilot-Induced Oscillation Tendencies of YF-12 Aircraft. Report No. NASA TN D-7900. Washington, D.C.: National Aeronautics and Space Administration.

[63]Smith, R. 1978. Effects of Control System Dynamics on Fighter Approach and Landing Longitudinal Flying Qualities (Vol. 1). Report No. AFFDL-TR-122. Wright-Patterson Air Force Base, Ohio: Air Force Flight Dynamics Laboratory.

[64]Smith, R. 1993. The Smith-Geddes Criteria. Presented at the SAE Aerospace, Control and Guidance Systems Symposium, Reno, Nevada, March 11, 1993. Mojave, California: High Plains Engineering.

[65]Smith, R. 1994. Predicting and Validating Fully-Developed PIO. AIAA Paper No. 94-3669. Pp. 1162-1166 in Proceedings of the AIAA Guidance, Navigation and Control Conference, Scottsdale, Arizona, August 1–3, 1994. Reston, Virginia: AIAA.

[66]Smith, R., and N. Geddes. 1979. Handling Quality Requirements for Advanced Aircraft Design: Longitudinal Mode. Report No. AFFDL-TR-78-154. Wright-Patterson Air Force Base, Ohio: Air Force Flight Dynamics Laboratory.
[67]Tischler, M.B., J.W. Fletcher, P.M. Morris, and G.E. Tucker. 1991. Flying quality analysis and flight evaluation of a highly augmented combat rotorcraft. Journal of Guidance, Control, and Dynamics 14(5):954–964.
[68]U.S. Army. 1994. Handling Qualities Requirements for Military Rotorcraft. ADS-33D. St. Louis, Missouri: U.S. Army Aviation and Troop Command.
[69]U.S. Department of Defense. 1980. Military Specification, Flying Qualities of Piloted Airplanes. MIL-F-8785C. Philadelphia, Pennsylvania: Department of Defense Military Specifications and Standards.
[70]U.S. Department of Defense. 1990. Department of Defense Interface Standard, Flying Qualities of Piloted Aircraft. MIL STD-1797A. Philadelphia, Pennsylvania: Department of Defense Military Specifications and Standards.
[71]U.S. Department of Defense. 1995. Department of Defense Interface Standard, Flying Qualities of Piloted Aircraft. MIL STD-1797A Update. Wright-Patterson Air Force Base, Ohio: Systems Engineering Division, Aeronautical Systems Center.